FITENOMICS
Your Health is Money

MR. RYAN WEBER

ISBN: 1478230657
ISBN 13: 9781478230656

Disclaimer

It is strongly advised that you consult with your physician before you start any kind of new health and fitness regimen. This book is not intended to diagnose, treat, or cure any physical ailments, diseases, or psychological conditions. As long as that is clear, may you enjoy the inspirational, motivational, and thought-provoking ideas presented in this book.

Special Thanks

I dedicate this book to God, first and foremost. Without God, none of this would have been possible. I offer a special thank you to all of my family, friends, and others who supported me during the writing of this book. It sometimes takes a little hard luck to discover what you are truly capable of accomplishing. Others can encourage you, but only you can take the action. If everything in life was meant to be easy, there would be no joy in your accomplishments. Ideas, inspiration, and guidance come from a wide array of people, experiences, and dreams. Thank you to all of those who have paved the way and made life's answers a little easier to discover along the way.

How To Use This Book

This book is intended for use as a guide on how to improve your overall health, wealth, fitness, and quality of life. It would be wise to read this book once all the way through and then refer back to different sections for clarity and purpose. The book is not particularly long, which makes it more digestible and easier for the reader to follow along. As a supplement to the book, visit http://www.fitenomics.com for further information and support about your health and fitness. For the latest up-to-the-minute updates be sure to follow us on Twitter@fitenomics and like us on Facebook. Best wishes to you in your quest for success and enjoyment that will last you a lifetime.

Table of Contents

Please, read this section before you start to read the rest of the book. This information is important for you to understand the ideas behind *Fitenomics*.

Preface

This is the confidence we have in approaching God: that if we ask anything according to his will, he hears us. And if we know that he hears us—whatever we ask—we know that we have what we asked of him.

— 1 JOHN 5 : 14 – 15
(N I V)

Do you remember the first fitness success book that you ever looked at? Maybe you read it; maybe you didn't. But was it something you could relate to? Could you relate to the author or the picture on the cover? When I first set out to publish this book, I wanted to make sure it had nothing to do with my personal story. I wanted this book to be about your journey into fitness, your goals, and your plan to get there safely and successfully. I worked very hard not to include myself in any of the writings because I did not want to cheapen the information. My thoughts were, *No one is going to care what I did to get in shape and build a successful life; they just want to know how to do it for themselves*. I wrote this way in order to eliminate any of the fluff, pats on the back, or egotistical undertones associated with self-proclaimed fitness gurus. I did not want to come off as a person who was overly satisfied with his accomplishments. This was meant to be your project, not mine.

Several people read the book and gave me their feedback; they all agreed there was something missing. From the writing, the reader didn't really know much about the author and how he came to his conclusions. After all, some of the ideas in this book stray far away from what some would call fitness based, but that was kind of the point. It may not be obvious, but most people should understand the sense of combining fitness with happiness, success, and relationships. This combined definition is going to be different for everyone, but it should still encompass the paradigm of self-help and self-improvement. A true sense of self-empowerment should be the overall outcome with a plan of how to get there safely—meaning, I do not want you to do anything you do not want to do; however, you should do the things that make you happy in life. If, in the process, you can refine your actions and make them that much better, then that is a good method to prove self-empowerment to yourself. You may not have been given the silver spoon in life, but you have the power to control what resources and thought patterns you are going to work with and how they will influence your life.

You already have a certain degree of leverage you can use to your benefit because you were the one to pick up this book. The change is in you; we just need to make sure we can express and support your progress the right way. The great thing about fitness is that it does come in different shapes and sizes. What is super fit and healthy for one person may not be the best way for you to do it. There are so many different nutrition plans and workouts available. It can get confusing as to who has the right plan of action for the best and most suitable results. The truth is that there is only one rule: there is nothing that will work 100 percent for everyone. A cookie-cutter fitness program is a great place to start, but the results will be different for everyone. No one person is built exactly like the next. There are trainers out there who get wonderful results over and over again, but they are not relying on training and nutrition alone. They have learned the concept of leverage and seek out clients who want to make a change and work very hard at it. Rome was not built in a day, and your physique will not be shaped in a day either. The people who come to them and use the methodology of health and fitness all have one thing in common: they came to make a change because they wanted to make a change. How they get there is important because they want to be safe while doing it, but it is not as relevant as the decision they made to make the change in the first place.

Youth and Experience

This may be a shocker to you, but I grew up a super-skinny kid. I was not overweight; I was underweight...and by quite a bit. Usually, you hear about the fat kid who was unpopular, got picked on, and had a totally miserable childhood. It wasn't until years later that I began to develop a bit of a chunky side, but we will talk about that later. The psychological problems that come with being too skinny are similar to those that accompany being too fat. To most people, skinny is a good thing, but it depends on how the word is used and reflected back to your peers. Some people were very genuine in saying, "I wish I were as skinny as you," while others said things to poke fun at me. The word *skinny* wasn't used as a compliment; it was used in a derogatory sense, along with related terms, like *Skeletor, AIDS patient, pencil neck, wimp, girly man, and ET*. These were some of the names I heard growing up. The ET slander was in reference to my neck being much thinner compared to the rest of my body. I remember one of my peers in grade school pointed to the back of my neck and said to me, "Dude, what is this? I think I can eat a bowl of cereal out of the back of your neck." I know this statement sounds ridiculous, but I was so skinny that when I when was leaning over my desk doing class work, it actually looked like my neck sank into my body. I'm laughing a bit now as I write this, but it wasn't so funny when I was younger.

The fact that I was so skinny proved to be an assumed weakness to the other kids at school. I was constantly a target for being picked on and beaten up. The funny thing was I wasn't too bad at holding my own. One-on-one fights didn't last too long because I was able to defend myself relatively well. It was when it turned into a group thing that it started to hurt and mess me up psychologically. Getting the crap pounded out of you by a group of your peers when you are trying to make it home for dinner just because they felt the urge is not an experience to be forgotten. I would fight back the best I could, but sometimes, it was overwhelming. My parents would see the bruises on my body and think I was a clumsy kid. I would explain to them I had gotten in a fight, but they had a hard time believing young kids could be so cruel. Don't get me wrong; my parents are awesome people, and they gave me everything they had. It was just an uncomfortable place to be in. It wasn't until one day when my father was picking me up early because I was sick and two kids were chasing me down in the parking lot that they understood. I was sick, and they still didn't give me a break even then. My father was visibly upset and apologized for the situation. It was not his fault; it was a case of kids being cruel because they were also hurting.

At that point, I began to fight back pretty hard. I felt like I could get away with a little more now that my parents knew what was happening. It is important to note that I did have quite a few friends growing up, but kids at the grade-school level were really weird about proving themselves. I don't know if they had jealousy issues or what. One day, I was a friend with a person, hanging out with him after school, and the next, we were beating each other up in the parking lot. Of course, when I would retaliate and fight back, that was when the teacher would look out the window and see me throwing the first punch. Then I would get in trouble at school, which would affect my studies, which then would get me in more trouble at home—continuing this cycle of frustration. It was a tough time to go through, but it made me stronger and who I am today.

When I first started high school, I felt like it was a new beginning. I was so excited to start over and not have to worry about grade school issues anymore. After all, high school was where the cooler and more mature kids went, right? After the honeymoon period of the first two months wore off, I was back where I started. Everyone else seemed to grow and put on weight while I stayed around a measly 115 pounds. I was about twenty pounds under most others in my class. Standing at almost five eleven, I was a beanpole. The trouble I got myself into in high school would probably fill a book in itself, and it did have an impact on my attitude, social interaction, grades, and confidence. The one thing that the teachers and some of the big football players would do was put their hands around my neck and steer me through the halls. I absolutely hated that! I knew I was skinny, but at this point, they were being domineering. I knew in my heart that someday, I was going to make a change and stick up for the kid who went through peer hell!

I could go on and on with more examples like these, but here is the point. You have the power to choose how you respond to any given experience. These experiences, as challenging as they were, made me who I am today. I don't reflect on the past and wish it could have been different. I use those experiences and leverage them into fuel for the fire. It inspires me to push myself and give life my best. It proves to me that adversity is in the eye of the beholder and that any situation can be turned into something positive. I don't let the thoughts of others influence who I am and what I am capable of. Life is not always going to be easy. Problems bring solutions, and the solutions you create for yourself may be the path that inspires many more people after you to go further and dig deeper when the outlook seems grim. What greater gift can you give someone—or yourself for that matter—than the gift of self-liberation? Knowing that no physical ailment or physical being can hold you down and prevent you from becoming what you really are is powerful. A real champion in life is someone who creates answers when none are to be found and opens doors that no one else looks for. It would have been too easy to just give up and give in, and I sure as heck was not going to do that!

Beginning a Career

When I graduated high school, I found time for a new hobby and passion—the gym. I was inspired to make a change in myself and the way other people saw me. I was going to do it for myself with the intention of proving to everyone I was not to be picked on any longer. I trained hard for several years and eventually gained quite a bit of muscle mass and weight. I ate as much food as I could and tried many different over-the-counter supplements, such as protein and creatine. I made very noticeable improvements and had people asking me all the time how to get in shape. A good friend at the time told me to write a book, but I just laughed at the idea—funny how things work out. I had a new passion in life at this point, and that was becoming a fireman/paramedic.

The testing process to get a full-time fire job is not easy. You need to attend the appropriate training at school and the academy, and then you have to test for a possible position with any given city that may be hiring. It can take up to several years even to be considered for a position. The first entrance exam I ever took was with two hundred other people. The test seemed to be easy, and I went in with a positive and confident attitude that I would score in the top five. About a month later, I finally got my results and was excited to see my accomplishment. I ended up placing 177 out of 200. My ego and hopes of getting hired quickly were squashed like a bug. It was quite a process to go through, and I was very grateful to get hired when I did.

The experiences I've had with the fire department through the years have greatly affected my outlook on life and the writing of this book. It is important to understand that anyone who works in the safety services—fire fighters, police officers, military service members, EMS medics—or in the medical field most likely has a stressful job. These men and women spend an enormous amount of time living and operating in the gray area of life and death. People do not call upon safety forces when they are having a good day; they call because they are in trouble, hurt, or helpless in some way. Our job is to quickly and efficiently mitigate a situation and provide some form of skill, relief, or comfort to help however possible. Our calls can range from something as minor as water leaks in a basement to a three-month-old baby who has stopped breathing.

We have had to deal with chronic alcoholics and heroin users who refuse to quit using and continuously get themselves into trouble. We become familiar with many patients who have a difficult time controlling their blood sugar only to show up one day when no one could get to them in time and find them dead on the floor. We spend countless nights with sick and diseased patients, witnessing the disease eat away at their minds and bodies. We spend the last few moments of people's lives with them when their family can't or don't care to. It can take its toll over time; however, it is the most rewarding feeling you can get when you have the opportunity to make someone's life that much better. We have talked to suicidal patients and gotten them help when no one would listen. We have brought back patients who were not breathing. We had one gentleman walk into the station and thank us three months later. We had a young woman who had been beaten by every significant male figure in her life find comfort in someone who took a minute to look her in the eyes and show her real compassion. These experiences can cause you to look at life very differently. Whenever you think you are having a bad day, remember there is always someone worse off than you. It is sad to think of it that way, but it is true.

Not everyone who is given a good bill of health takes care of him- or herself. There are many patients we see on a weekly basis who continue to have the same problems. However, we also see patients who try to do everything right and still suffer from disease and ailments. Your life and health are gifts and should be treated as such. If you were born healthy and have the opportunity to live a productive and meaningful life, you should do it. If anything, do it for the people who are crippled by disease and never have the opportunity to experience what you may take for granted. If you are already living a healthy and happy life, I am super excited for you, and I thank you for valuing yourself. You never know whom you may help and inspire along the way.

Health and fitness mean something different for everyone. If you eat well, feel good, and exercise but still drink alcohol on the weekends, you are trying much harder than the drug addict or very obese person who doesn't care about him- or herself. It is one thing to feel discouraged if you are making an effort and not seeing the results you want compared to a person who blatantly throws his or her life in the toilet with drugs or eats so much food that he or she weighs over four hundred pounds. Guess what; we take them to the hospital too. It is very difficult trying to get a four-hundred-fifty-pound male or female out of the house when they call 911. It is very often this type of person who will say they cannot walk on their own and needs to be carried. Even if you have six in-shape firemen trying to bring this person down the stairs through a small and cluttered hallway, it's still very challenging. The patient may become offended when it takes so much manpower, but what can we realistically do with these people? Someone is going to get hurt, which puts us in danger along with the patient. If you think I am making this up, by all means please, ask another fire fighter, medic, nurse, doctor, police officer, etc., and hear what he or she has to say about it. These are all real situations I have had to deal with at work.

With that being said, I have a different outlook on what health and fitness means to the public. All of these experiences can evoke a certain type of passionate response in a fit, health-conscious person. Drug addicts' lack of respect for themselves and the constant complaining they provide about how their life is horrible all the way to the hospital can be a bit much. The people doing all the complaining are the only ones who can make a change. Believe me; I'm rooting for them all the way because their lives are a gift and should be treated as such.

My hope is that none of the content in this book is too harsh or too blunt, but I will not try to sugarcoat anything and make it less than what it is. That would not be fair to someone who is honest about making a change or wants to keep a good thing going. Keep in mind that if something triggers an emotional response in you, you should pay attention to it. That is passion expressing itself in the finest light. Embrace what your passions are telling you, and use them to respond in the most useful way possible. Your passions and emotional responses are the triggers for making a change. Get to know them well, and understand that change is not easy and it may even hurt. Stick with it, and it will pay off in the end. God put the desire in your heart for a reason.

Human Capital

A book called *Naked Economics* by Charles Wheelan was published in 2002. In it, he gives a very good definition of what human capital is. He defines human capital as "the sum total of skills embodied within an individual: education, intelligence, charisma, creativity, work experience, entrepreneurial vigor, and even the ability to throw a baseball fast. It's what you would be left with if someone striped away all of your assets—your job, your money, your home, your possessions—and left you on the street corner with only your clothes." In my opinion, this definition should also encompass the idea of health and fitness.

Human capital is the end result of what we are made of. It is what our successes and failures are built upon. It is what this country and this world were built upon. If you lack the ability, the drive, the desire, the skills, and the intestinal fortitude to build a worthwhile and successful life, you essentially lack human capital. A poor life, a poor attitude, poor health, and poor fitness are symptoms of a lack of human capital. The good news is that these are all within your power to change and do something about. Your overall quality of life is in direct proportion to your personal level of health and fitness. Your personal relationships, your business relationships, your attitude, and your outlook are all affected at the physical and subconscious levels.

Choices

The choices you make now about your health and fitness are going to affect your and your family's future in a large way. Your persona, your accomplishments, your confidence, your appearance, your sex appeal, your thought processes and judgments, your career, your income, your insurance costs, and your longevity on this earth are a just a few examples. No one can say exactly in what way or how you will be affected, just know that you will. Here are a few ideas to consider: someone who is more aesthetically pleasing demonstrates survival of the fittest or a strong mating partner. Our whole culture and existence revolves around evolution, and your fitness will allow you to meet a more quality partner. Someone who is in better shape and takes care of him- or herself demonstrates to an employer he or she has a strong work ethic. A better-positioned job equates to more income and job potential. Someone who eats a healthier selection of foods will have more energy, healthier blood pressure and cholesterol levels, and clearer thought processes. A clearer thought process will help you to see and understand that luck is opportunity in disguise. Someone who exercises has an outlet for stress and is less likely to harbor feelings of hurtfulness and anxiety. A calm sense of oneself is an admirable leadership trait. The list can go on and on as to how the benefits of choosing and investing in your own health and well-being are beneficial.

You may be one of the fortunate individuals who already live a rich life in the monetary sense. Money definitely does make life easier, but it will not lead to complete happiness. Just because you have money does not mean you also possess the decency and self-respect so many desire. There are several lost souls who can be handed whatever they believe will make them happy and still feel empty. Life is not something that happens to you; you happen to it. Time will go on with or without you. There is a deep human desire to feel we have earned something on our own. There are many lazy people in the world who would rather sit on a couch and collect a check; I have met several of them. That does not mean they are actually happy; they are just coasting on the easy and meaningless way out. I hope and pray that people who are that lost see the light one day and make a change for the better. Life is much bigger than oneself, and the one who helps his or her fellow man get what he or she wants will be much more fulfilled and understand true wealth and happiness.

You have to earn your health and well-being, period. There is no way around that. You can't just take a pill to create the ultimate physique and quality of fitness you want. Keeping your body healthy, or working hard to be in the best shape possible is in essence answering life's call to earn the respect and feeling of accomplishment so many want. It is honoring yourself, your fellow man, and God. It is the gateway to achieving whatever you want to achieve in life. It is inspiration at its finest. I hope you were born healthy and do not suffer from any diseases or ailments. Even if one was born with or acquired a disease or disability, one should still try to achieve his or her own best health state.

Fitness Is Dynamic

I mentioned that I started out super skinny. Over the years of eating to put on size and muscle, I did get to a point where I started to get a little chubby around the waistline. I was working in my parents' yard when someone made a comment about my "love handles." It didn't register at first, but then I recalled person after person who would say to me, "Just wait, you will start to put on weight like the rest of us." The person who told me I was getting love handles had a smile ear to ear. It was like this person was so happy to see I was entering that state of physical condition. If you are one of those people waiting to say, "I told you so," to someone who may have lost his or her way, get a life! Instead of waiting for someone to fall to a less than desirable level, you should adopt an attitude of growth and maturity and help that person stay on track. It is a sign of maturity to grow and work to encourage people rather than belittle them.

I was very fortunate when I first began working out to have a friend who showed me how and what to do in the gym for the first five years. He trained me almost every day and never asked for a dime. We became good friends, and because of his commitment to me, he and the gym were what kept me out of a lot of trouble my peers got into after high school. It was a very crucial point in my life. I may never have gotten my fireman job if I had not started working out and kept away from troublesome people. I may have really gotten tied up with the peer pressure and made some poor decisions. I am forever grateful and will always appreciate what that man did for me and what he did for several other young men at our gym. He was an excellent role model and gave much of himself so that many others would benefit from his knowledge and experience. He has since passed on, but he will never be forgotten. Thank you very much, Mr. Donald DeVito.

As I am writing this book, I am currently competing in men's physique competitions across the country. I am not writing this to brag or encourage you to do the same; I mention it because it has changed my life for the better. I have always had the dream to be on a competitive fitness level, but I was scared to do it. I was afraid that I might not be good enough and would be laughed at. Since I have stopped caring about what other people may think, competition has given me something to look forward to and focus positive attention on. I used to look forward to getting drunk every weekend and partying my youth away. Sure, it was fun for a while, but I was beginning to feel very empty inside. I was beginning to develop a form of depression I did not know how to express or relate to anyone. I was also starting to get love handles! Now that I am working very hard to excel in one aspect of life, I feel as though I am reaping the benefits across the board. When you reach for success in one area of your life, it tends to spill over into other areas. More important, stepping outside of the box and chasing a dream others thought you would not be capable of is very inspiring to many people.

Be Thankful

Because of the support of my family, friends, and co-workers, I have been very fortunate to experience an opportune life thus far. I am very excited to see just how far I can take it and how many people I can help and inspire along the way. It was and always has been about something much bigger than personal accomplishments. It is about inspiring a positive change in people and the lives they live. Fitness is the vehicle to take you from where you are right now to where you really want to be. God willing, it is the first of many more blessings to come.

While you may assume health is common and take it for granted, this is not the case for everyone. I was extremely fortunate to do an interview with a very bright, positive, and grateful woman when I visited California on vacation. She is happily married with a beautiful son. In her interview, she talked about how her son has had to deal with health issues since birth. She explained how she, her husband, and her son work as a team to get the most out of life, health, and passion. Afraid that she had told me too much, she was concerned about whether I should post the interview or not. After she talked it over with her family and gave me her response, I will never forget the reason she said to go ahead with the publication. In her son's words, she said, "It is my mom's responsibility to teach people how lucky they are to have their bodies, and I am totally OK with it." This touched me in a way I cannot fully explain. If a young boy can be that understanding and have the foresight to see the positive side of a situation that can be viewed differently, he forever has my respect. I feel it is my job now more than ever to share with people how they can use health and fitness to create the life they dream of. Please take the time to view the video here http://www.fitenomics.com/interviews/. I hope it will touch your heart as it did mine. Thank you very much to the Hendershot family. You are an inspiration!

This book is walking the walk and talking the talk. I hope to address real-life concerns many face that other books did not address. It is written from a different perspective pertaining to a fast-paced, time-limited, and largely gray area of life, witnessing the dark and light side of human action, interaction, and real-life circumstances. My time as a fireman/paramedic has been well spent helping many people over the years. It is my hope to help many more in the years to come. It was and always has been a team effort with my co-workers, friends, and patients. No man or woman is an island in this business; we constantly rely on each other to get the job done. Please keep an open mind and take the time to reflect on all of your life's blessings thus far. I hope you enjoy *Fitenomics: Your Health Is Money*.

PHAT Introduction

Please Help, Advise, and Teach

It is every person's responsibility to help one another be the best they can be. It is better to build up those around you than bring them down. Everyone is connected in some fashion, and if one goes down, all will suffer.

—RYAN WEBER

The Cold, Hard Reality

How many successful fat people do you know? Even better, how many fat people do you know who are rich and famous? Actors, singers, models, and athletes are usually in good shape. When it comes to the general population, however, obesity is fairly close to mainstream. According to the *Obesity Research Journal*, statistics show that about 33 percent of the population maintains a healthy weight. This means that about two-thirds of the population is at an unhealthy weight. Around 33 percent of the US population is obese, and 67 percent is overweight. Statistics can always change, but this is an alarming number of overweight individuals.

When you go to the doctor for a checkup, the nurse usually has you stand on a scale. Doctors use a chart that lists specific weight ranges based on your height to diagnose if you're overweight. If you do not fall in the recommended category, you are considered to be over-or-underweight. Since people come in all different shapes and sizes, it is probably safe to assume this chart is not 100 percent accurate. However, the small number of people who the chart does not properly represent will not make up for the larger percentage who the chart accurately reflects. Athletes, odd-balls, and midgets alike will not be enough to tip the scale in favor of being incorrect. This means that the original 67 percent estimation is somewhere in the ballpark of being correct. So what does this mean to you? Do you fall into the larger and more unfit category, or are you in the smaller, healthy category?

The word "fat" is not a very pleasant term to use. It is rather crude and kind of mean. Better and more politically correct terms to use may be "obese" and "overweight." Although all of these terms are used in this text, the word "fat" has a different emphasis on it. It doesn't sound very nice when it rolls off the tip of your tongue. Its unpleasant and abrupt sound is supposed to tell you something. It should help you realize that being fat or unhealthy is not a pleasant state to be in. If society were to keep coddling you and trying not to hurt your feelings by using politically correct terminology, you would have no reason to change. It's as if society is saying, "Hey, it's all right that you're fat and out of shape. We will just make nicer words and more excuses for you, so you don't feel as bad." Is that the right thing to do? Probably not! That is what helped get society into trouble in the first place.

This is not meant to be a personal attack on your ego, but it can be difficult to hear. By no means should you limit your self-worth due to a number on the scale. You should, however, ask yourself whether you are truly happy or not. If the answer eludes you or leaves you with something more to be desired, simply reflect on what it is you want to feel, lift your head high, and start living your life like you are the best self you can be. Do not wait; do it now, with no hesitation or delay. If you have previously made excuses in your life as to why you have not done something the instant you thought of it, you should realize that the time to enact your personal power and change is now.

This is a call to action. You can get upset if you feel the need to, but how is that going to help the situation get any better? There are tons of resources to help you get and stay healthy. They most likely will not fall out of the sky into your lap. You may have to go looking for help. The good news is that help is not that far away. Take advantage of the support systems and wealth of knowledge that are available to help you achieve a healthier lifestyle. This will directly impact your level of financial success, as well. Your overall health and fitness go hand in hand with your money and earning potential. If you take charge of your future now, you can provide a wealthy and prosperous life for you and your family to enjoy for a long time.

How Many Old Fat People Do You Know?

Many of the world's highly successful people are very mature in age. They didn't get this way from being fat and out of shape; they took care of themselves. Overweight people usually don't live long enough to enjoy wealth and prosperity at the higher level. Their health problems lead to a poor quality of life and stand in the way of their progress. The obese population has a greater number of health issues and higher mortality rates. It's obvious that people who don't take care of their health die at a younger age. Does this mean that your level of fitness and overall health can be directly related to the amount of money you earn? If obese people did live as long as the healthier crowd, they would probably stand a greater chance of reaching the upper ranks of monetary success. Having a healthy mind and body and a strong work ethic is a better recipe for success than being overweight and lazy.

The idea of wealth isn't just about money; it also includes your health. What good is being wealthy and successful if you can't enjoy it? Sure, you can do your family a huge monetary favor and leave behind a boatload of cash, but you should be able to enjoy the fruits of your labor. Many people act like it's a joke that they are overweight and aren't going to be around as long as expected. It's a ridiculous concept that doesn't make much sense to them, though some of these overweight individuals are really just trying to hide from the fact they're afraid of what might happen. Not many are ready and willing to openly face criticism without using humor as a shield to hide behind. They may even barricade themselves to such an extent that they go into denial. It's very difficult to reason with people who *know* they are right without any exception.

There usually is an exception to every rule. It is said that, "You should never believe anything too much, because there will always be a situation where it is not true." This may be a good philosophy to live by, but what if it is true? Then you are going to look stupid for not believing it. You were given a mind to use with the hopes of not wasting it. Exercise your opinions, and make decisions for yourself. There are some very successful obese people in the world who get so caught up in their success, they just forget about their health. They still make a lot of money, drive a nice car, have a big house, take vacations, and are wonderful people. However, they also have more handicaps than healthier people do, such as high blood pressure, high cholesterol, difficulty breathing, lack of suitable public accommodations, higher health and life insurance costs, and shorter life spans. After all, true beauty is on the inside but, it is something to think about.

If you're still having some doubts about this obesity thing, think of the last time you sat next to a grossly overweight person. Could you hear the person breathing and struggling for oxygen? Maybe he or she was holding a bottle of oxygen in order to survive a trip outside of the house. This is an extreme example but, people who need to use oxygen tanks during the day probably have to sleep with a breathing machine at night. Do you think these people pay for the oxygen and breathing machines themselves? If they don't pay for them, who does? Are they covered by insurance? Have you ever stopped and thought about how much this costs the insurance companies? If you haven't, you are now. This may even be costing you money out of your own pocket. These issues will be discussed in more detail later on in the book.

Choice Is an Option, Not a Command

So what can you do right now to change the grim outlook of your future if you are overweight? For starters, you need to admit it. After that, the answer is simple: eat well, think well, and exercise. If you do these three things, your chances of living a more prosperous, successful, happy, and fulfilled life are much greater. Telling yourself it doesn't matter to anyone else except you is a very dumb and selfish statement. You most likely have a family to consider. Your wife, husband, or kids are counting on you to be there and support them. They want you to love them, teach them, and help them when they are in need. They would do it for you if the situation were reversed. Your mother, father, sister, brother, grandma, and grandpa all want the best for you. They want you to grow and leave behind a strong family legacy. How would they feel if you just gave up on yourself? How would you truly feel if you gave up on yourself? Since you are reading this, you're probably not a quitter. Now it's time for you to prove it.

So many people in your life have invested time in you. Family, friends, teachers, coworkers, and maybe even strangers have had an impact in your life and development. Honor their time and commitment with you, no matter how short or long it may have been, and prove to yourself that you're a winner. Maybe you had a rough childhood and your family didn't support you. Maybe you were the type who didn't have very many friends growing up. It's time to quit making excuses and feeling sorry for yourself. You can't let past experiences haunt you and predict your future. The outcome of your life is up to you, and the decisions you make are your own. Take responsibility for your actions, and quit putting the blame on someone else. Choice is an option, not a command. You have the power to choose what you're going to get out of this life. If you choose wisely, you will be much happier with the decisions you make.

Think of all the people who have gone before you who wish they had the opportunity to make a difference. Maybe they felt they were not given a fair chance at life, and maybe they have a whole bunch of other excuses to hide the fact they never tried hard enough. Ask yourself these five questions, and do your best to answer them honestly:

1. How can I become a better and more able person?
2. Are the obstacles in front of me so great that there is no way to overcome them?
3. If given the solution to my problem, would I be willing to apply it?
4. Why do I want to change?
5. Who do I want to become?

Sometimes you need to do a little soul searching to figure out what you really want. Things change, and what was important to you yesterday may not be today.

Fulfillment

Fulfillment is measured differently by everyone. Do you know what fulfillment is for you? For you, enjoying happiness might mean that you are fulfilled. To someone else, it might be about being successful. What about your freedom? Having the ability to be free and do whatever you want can be a form of fulfillment. While achieving any one of these three goals— happiness, success, and freedom—would be nice, perhaps true fulfillment involves achieving all three in conjunction with each other. Maybe fulfillment is really a kind of self-awareness.

In other words, maybe reaching all three of these desired levels of awareness are necessary to form a balance. It should make sense to you that everything in life is dependent on a type of balance. Your body relies on its pH balance to be in the healthy range, the ecological system is dependent upon balance in the environment, and the solar systems are balanced throughout the universe. In order for your life to be as success-ful as it can be, you must maintain a balance.

For example, if you want to increase your physical health and success, you need to study and increase your mental capacity, as well. Reading books, taking a class, and putting into practice what you have learned will require some thinking and planning on your part. In order to increase your mental capacity, you need to find the means to do so. You also have to increase your social success. You need to talk to people to find out where the information is that will help you improve your level of fitness. Unless you were born with all the answers, talking to people who have knowl-edge to share will give you a better chance at being successful and accomplishing your goal. Improving yourself in one area will help you to improve in other areas.

Is This Your Problem or Your Opportunity?

Remember the movie *The Matrix*? It is a futuristic thriller about fighting for the rights of humanity in a virtual reality. There is a part in the movie where the lead actor, Keanu Reeves, is given the choice between living in reality (the red pill) and living in perceived reality (the blue pill). Ultimately, he chooses to take the red pill, thereby wiping out all of life's perceived reality. The truth becomes evident and is very difficult for Reeves to swallow. The same goes for you. The truth can hurt if you are not ready for it. Right now you may be realizing what the real truth is about your health and level of fiscal security. It is not always what you expect it to be. Now that the idea has been planted in your mind, it will continue to grow. Your perceptions of truth and reality are being challenged to create a more meaningful and abundant life for you and your family.

You were meant to live a wealthy and prosperous life. In order for you to enjoy it to the fullest extent, you need to be sure that your health is up to par. Your precious time and money will be wasted if you decide to ignore this truth. You need to wake up and take hold of what is yours in this world. Do not let the preconceived notion of "it's not your fault" ruin and run your life. It will end up costing you way too much in the end.

The Cost to Society

Do you know how much money is spent on obese and out-of-shape people in the United States? A news release from the Society of Actuaries, published on January 10, 2011, stated that the estimated amount spent on obesity in the United States and Canada was 300 billion dollars. America was responsible for $270 billion, while Canada was only responsible for $30 billion. Here is the breakdown that was included in the release:

- Increased need for medical care: $127 billion
- Loss of worker productivity due to higher rates of death: $49 billion
- Loss of productivity due to loss of productive workers: $43 billion
- Loss of productivity due to total disability: $72 billion

These are staggering numbers. Where do you think this money is coming from? Sure, you're not handing it to them directly, but your health-care providers and insurance companies are. Maybe this is why health insurance costs are rising and companies are cutting benefits. Big business does not want to spend money on people who do not take care of themselves.

Who can blame them? The Society of Actuaries also released the results from an online survey of a thousand people. Of those who responded, 83 percent said they would consider a healthy lifestyle alternative if there was some sort of an incentive from the insurance companies. Really? Well that is good to know. All you have to do is throw some more money at the overstuffed population, and they will consider a change. How is that for a remedy?

What Does This Really Cost You?

Think for a moment of all the things in life that you enjoy and may take for granted. Materialistic things like a nice house, new car, stylish clothes, and extravagant vacations may come to mind. Now think of all of the things that really matter to a human being—things like family, meeting and falling in love with your significant other, raising your children, taking your daughter to her first dance, and watching your son play his favorite sport. These are the real treasures you risk giving up when you do not take care of your health and fitness. Your well-being is not just yours anymore when you have a family; it is something you are all invested in.

From a monetary standpoint, you might be wondering what it costs to join a gym and eat healthier food. You might believe you will have to spend a little extra in order to get into shape. First of all, this would be a horrible way to look at things. Your health and wellness are invaluable, and to put a price on them is ridiculous. The small amount of money you may spend on a gym membership is nothing compared to what you will spend on health care if you don't take care of yourself, not to mention the cost of missing out on life's love and memories should you become handicapped by obesity. Neglect will be the thing that costs you, not your workouts.

It is easy to make excuses as to why you cannot do something. It is as if you have a special circumstance that no one else can understand except you. No one else has the same reality checks that you do. You have a litany of excuses: you have to wake up early for work, you did not get much sleep last night, you got sick, you have to work late, you have homework to do, you have an appointment you cannot miss, the kids take up all your time, your wife or husband wants to see you more, you did not feel like it, and something came up. While these are all great excuses, they do not separate you from the rest of the normal and functioning people in the world. They all have the same obstacles, but they deal with them and still get things handled. They take care of their health and fitness while balancing family, work, school, the big game, guys and ladies night, unexpected circumstances, and life in general. You must maintain a healthy balance in your life.

Think about the people in this world who really have been given the short end of the stick—people who were born into war, poverty, disease, and misfortune and who live in the slums in underdeveloped countries. They did not ask for that kind of a life but have to deal with it anyway. Without any thought whatsoever, many of these less fortunate people wake up and function on a daily basis. They may be considered poor and sick, but given the chance to do something greater and the knowledge that they truly have the potential to be loved and are rich in heart and spirit, any one of these people would be glad to live the life many people take for granted and say is too stressful and busy. They would not waste an opportunity to live healthy and happy lives.

Realize you have been given the opportunity so many wish they can have. Be grateful and do not take for granted the gift you wake up with each morning. Share your gifts with the world, and use them to make your own life better. In the process you will be honoring those around you who wish to go in the same positive direction and will make their lives better. Your actions can and might be the one positive influence that helps change someone else's life. You never know who is watching and what that person is capable of. Maybe all that people need to hear is that they are special and were born with the gift to live and grow into greatness. Maybe if they saw you expressing gratitude for your gifts, they would be able to imagine themselves doing the same. Your enthusiasm and determination to live better, stronger, and healthier can now be the seed that grows in someone else's mind. You can share with them the same gift you were given. When you look at it from this standpoint, you'll see that what you have to lose can be very great. This doesn't necessarily have to be money; in fact, it may be more of an idea. The intangibles in life can sometimes cost you dearly if you do not pay attention. The next time your spouse, son, or daughter smiles at you, be aware of the power that is behind that smile. You have the opportunity to share something great with your loved ones that they can share with the whole world. And all of this can come from a simple idea of including fitness with your health and happiness. Train for your fitness, enjoy your happiness, and share your results with the world.

Millennium Development Goals

The idea behind the Millennium Development Goals (MDG) is to help bring underdeveloped countries up to speed with the rest of the developed world. For example, poor countries like India need help decreasing the level of poverty there. The HIV/AIDS epidemic that haunts Africa and other poorly developed locations needs to be addressed. Something as basic as establishing a primary system of education in poor countries also merits attention. With an education system in place, people could be taught how to protect themselves from diseases, which would be a huge step in the right direction. Healthy and educated individuals have a better chance at making a good life for themselves.

These goals were accepted by the United Nations back in 2000. The member countries hope to have these problems under control by 2015. Over half of the target concepts that make up the Millennium Development Goals have to do with improving one's health. It is understood that the people living in these countries do not have a good chance of improving unless they can establish a strong healthy baseline. Health combined with education will provide the foundation for success—in other words, wealth. Establishing a solid nutrition plan, complete with a fitness training regimen, is a great place to start.

From a logistics standpoint, achieving these goals will require a massive amount of resources. Every man, woman, and child able to contribute will help the cause. But who will take the responsibility for making sure this happens? When everyone agrees to be involved and is on board, it is easy to wait for someone else to step up and take charge. If everyone assumes that someone else is in charge, each person is simply waiting to be called upon for help. If no one does step up, then the goals are not going to be reached and the problem will continue to grow.

Getting back to the problem at hand, the obesity crisis is a problem that conveys the same feelings of responsibility on a smaller scale. Everyone knows it is a problem and claims to be on board to fix it, but the problem remains an enigma. Who will step up and take the lead in working toward a healthy and fit world? It only takes one to start the cascade of leadership. That one person who can begin to make a difference is you. The sooner that fitness becomes a part of your life, the sooner you can begin to enjoy the rewards it has to offer and share them with others.

Now It's Up to You

Think about yourself for a moment. Do you know what your short-term goals are? Do have you any long-term goals in place? If not, you need to do this now! Take responsibility for your life and establish your goals. Think about what your needs and desires are and how you can go about getting them. Take action now. The moment you do, you will begin to see some positive changes. Life is full of forks in the road, and the decisions you make right now will echo throughout the rest of your existence on this planet. Realize you have the power to establish and fulfill whatever role you want in life; no matter how large or how small, it is yours for the taking.

You should have your own Millennium Development Goals and challenge others to do the same. It should be a necessity that you think bigger than yourself and stretch your potential. There are so many alternatives for you to choose from to live a healthier and happier life. This book is a tool to help improve your everyday self. Start using it today and continue using it tomorrow and for the rest of your life to become a better person. Ten years from now, you can still refer to this book and see how it has changed and inspired you.

How a Champion Is Born

Choosing to be positive and having a grateful attitude is going to determine how you're going to live your life.

— JOEL OSTEEN

Imagine you are a young boy from a small town near Graz in Austria. You come from a hardworking and honest family struggling to make ends meet. You realize at a young age you are going to want more from life and begin to dream of what could be. Not many will agree with your dreams, and some will even tell you that they are not possible. You are told your current situation will never allow for something life changing and great to happen. How will you be able to accomplish all of these wonderful ideas you have if no one believes in you? The answer is that you will have to rely on your own strength and determination to be successful.

After being introduced to sports, you begin to see the bigger picture. What if you can be better than everyone else and climb your way to the top? If you work to become a physically dominant individual, train hard, and gain world recognition, you could possibly make all of your dreams come true. You realize that physical fitness can be the vehicle to take you where you want to go in life. After hours, days, and years of hard work, your fitness lifestyle will pay off big-time. This is the kind of mindset that led champion bodybuilder Arnold Schwarzenegger to become the greatest of his kind in a physically spectacular sport.

Arnold's father introduced him to sports at a young age to help teach him discipline. After playing several sports, Arnold realized his true passion was with the sport of bodybuilding. He began to compete at the age of fifteen and steadily climbed his way to the top of an emerging and cinematic sport. He had the dream of being recognized as the best and would stop at nothing to achieve his goal. He knew he was going to have a successful career, and there wasn't anything that could stand in his way.

Bodybuilding Beginning

Bodybuilding is a competitive sport in which you lift weights and practice excellent nutrition to create a physique that demonstrates symmetry, muscular definition, size, and power. There are many levels of the sport, most notably the International Federation of Bodybuilding and Fitness (IFBB). This is the category that interests so many and draws a large following. Many of the larger competitions will feature IFBB competitors as the main attraction.

With the explosive premiere of *Pumping Iron* on January 18, 1977, the sport of bodybuilding was introduced to the public at large. Arnold Schwarzenegger was showcased as the undefeated bodybuilding champion of the world. Although he had already retired from the sport of bodybuilding, he was convinced to train one last time for the Mr. Olympia competition so that the training and lifestyle of a competitive bodybuilder could be filmed for a movie. The movie helped introduce the charm, character, and charisma he displayed as a young athlete. His drive for success and uncompromising discipline proved to pay off in a larger-than-life kind of way.

He went on to have a successful career in the movie business and became one of the biggest Hollywood box office stars ever. His first small break was in a film called *Hercules in New York*, which was released in 1970. In 1977, the documentary drama *Pumping Iron* was released and showcased his personality and character to the world. In 1982, he made *Conan the Barbarian*, which was a huge success and grossed a hundred million dollars at the box office. He was now making a big name for himself as an actor. His biggest break came when he starred in the hit action movie *The Terminator*, in which he played one of Hollywood's biggest and most terrifying villains ever. His muscular and massive physique helped to launch his career to an extraordinary level.

Education

While staying competitive during his bodybuilding career, Arnold received a business degree from the University of Wisconsin. His discipline began in athletics but was carrying over to other parts of his life. He wanted to be successful and knew that getting an education was important. He received his degree in business while still competing in bodybuilding competitions.

Arnold made several good investments that have paid off handsomely. He started his business ventures back when he was still competing in bodybuilding and continues working on them today. The discipline he developed playing sports and lifting weights has been leading his successful career every step of the way.

Opportunities

Arnold was able to capitalize on his successful career in bodybuilding with some related business ventures. He used his knowledge of the sport to write the two-volume *Encyclopedia of Bodybuilding*. He also wrote *The Education of a Bodybuilder*, which did very well.

His successful movie career allowed him to further expand his efforts. He believed in giving back to the community and, more important, investing in today's youth. He began an after-school program called the After-School All Stars to keep kids off the streets and out of trouble. He was appointed chairman of the President's Council on Physical Fitness and Sports and served in that capacity for three years. He was even asked to carry the torch in the 2002 Olympics. His accomplishments have been many and great. Even with his busy schedule, he continues to push forward and make new goals for himself.

Present Day

After all of these ventures, Arnold is still fueled by his fitness-based lifestyle. He was the governor of California and remains a powerful political figure. His accomplishments from bodybuilding and the movie business are still alive and well today in his political career. From marketing himself to promoting his ideas and values, Arnold Schwarzenegger is a living example of what a healthy lifestyle can provide to an individual who takes fitness seriously.

Each year, he holds a sports festival and competition in Columbus, Ohio, known as the Arnold Classic. During his body-building career, he visited Columbus for an event and was blown away by how well received the sport was. When he decided to host the sports festival on a yearly basis, Columbus became his location of choice. Now his fitness-based event attracts over a hundred and fifty thousand people each year and is still growing. How about that for an economic stimulus! The businesses, com-petitors, and spectators flood the city for four days just to catch a glimpse of what fitness can do for them. Even though Arnold keeps a busy schedule, he still finds time to visit and support the event he started. The Arnold Classic has immortalized his body-building career and has helped him reach icon status.

In a past article about then-Governor Schwarzenegger in *Muscle and Fitness* magazine, one of his staff members said that his energy level was still very high. The staffer noted that he had more energy and accomplished more with his day early in the morning than most people half his age did. His staff fed off of his energy and drive to make things happen and be more productive. His enthusiasm is a strong point, as it was in his competitive days. The discipline he learned from becoming a champion many years earlier is just as evident today.

There Will Be Many More

There have been many individuals who have made a great name for themselves in the interest of health and fitness. It may have started with fitness but definitely did not end there. Fitness is simply a gateway goal that, once achieved, can be developed into a lifetime of prosperity, happiness, and good fortune. The name Arnold Schwarzenegger is now synonymous with muscles, fitness, and success. Mr. Schwarzenegger has built an empire and made himself a household name. He is living proof of what you can be if you apply yourself and live a fitness-based lifestyle.

Your health is a wonderful gift that should not be taken for granted. If you have your health, you should be very grateful that you have been given the chance to be anything or anyone you want to be. Take this opportunity to ask yourself what you want your life to be like. Only you know the answer and have the power to do anything about it. You never know if you will be the next big thing. In fact, it is up to you to decide that you are going to be the next big thing and to go for it!

The Six Rules of Success

Visit www.fitenomics.com/motivation and you'll see a video summarizing a speech that Arnold once gave about his six rules of success. The rules are:

1. Trust yourself.
2. Break some rules.
3. Don't be afraid to fail.
4. Don't listen to the naysayers.
5. Work your butt off.
6. Give something back.

The video is only four minutes and twenty-six seconds long and is very inspiring. This is a small investment of your time that can make a huge difference in your attitude and outlook for the future.

A Sign of the Times

"You don't have to be great to start, but you have to start to be great."

—Zig Ziglar

It is never too late to start living a healthy and fit lifestyle. If you do not want to lift weights, you can use your body and some other handy devices to execute your resistance training program at home. If running or walking is more your style, you can visit the local parks or go to the gym and use the equipment. No matter where you live or what the weather may be like outside, you always have several options at your disposal. Before you know it, fitness will become second nature to you and you will not have to think much about what you are going to do to stay healthy. You'll just do it! Scheduling your workouts, planning your meals, and prioritizing your time are tasks that will become part of your everyday routine. If you are not already doing this, it may be hard to imagine what such a lifestyle would be like. You need to imagine what it would be like, formulate the ideas and images in your mind, and set out to create your new physically dominant reality.

Getting started can be one of the most difficult things to do. It is so easy to say to yourself and everyone else that you are going to start something. Whether they believe you or not depends on your character and previous claims you have made. If you have not followed through in the past, now is a great time to start and see what you are made of. This is the time to identify your reasons for becoming more of a healthy, fit, and motivated person. This decision will not only impact your health in a positive way but will also have a positive effect on your social, professional, and personal life. Better relationships, better sex, and more money should make anyone's self confidence shoot through the roof. Feeling good is contagious. When you are really clear about what you want and why, things will begin to happen that will shape the outcome of your future forever. Pretty soon you will have people approaching you and asking how they can transform themselves as you have. There is no greater compliment than being approached by someone who admires the commitment and dedication you display. Maybe you will even be the next guru and will inspire those around you to do the same.

Many people allow age to be the determining factor for whether they are able to get into shape or not. What the mind perceives the body believes, and you will not be able to move past your perception of reality until you change your mind-set. Before you can take on any new endeavor, you need to make sure you are thinking clearly. Your fitness level does not depend on your age. The more aware you are of your health and the harder you train, the better chance you have of making yourself appear years younger. By eating the right foods and exercising on a regular basis, you give yourself the advantage of slowing the aging process and living a more productive life. On the other hand, if you are out of shape and get back into shape, you can reverse the damage you caused by years of unhealthy living. This is as close to the fountain of youth as you can get. It is not a single food you eat or action you take that will bring you positive results, but rather a collection of sound and healthy practices.

As with any goal you set out to achieve, there are going to be obstacles you face along the way. The obstacles that stand in front of your success are going to be unique to your situation. It is up to you to put in the work and dedication to remove those obstacles. You may find that by removing one obstacle, you are able to improve other areas in your life that may have been previously suppressed.

This can be challenging, however. If it were that easy to remove adversities from your life, everyone would do it. Gracefully transitioning yourself into a "better you" requires a sense of pride and a willingness to make an effort. Sometimes the things you want in life need to be a bit more difficult to obtain so you can appreciate them more. You do need to be challenged. Your diligence and personal touch make the reward more meaningful; that way there is more value attached to the outcome and more of a reason to keep it in high regard. It is kind of like saying that without sadness there can be no happiness. You need to feel the difference before you can see the real value; otherwise everything would be relatively boring and stay the same. Once you recognize and desire the reward it's worth your time and effort.

If you do not have reason enough for improving your health, you need to create a "why" for yourself. Developing and coming up with a "why" will give you a huge advantage over someone who just goes through the motions. A person with a "why" is an individual with a plan for how to accomplish a goal. Many people go to work every day without really knowing why they are there. They may claim that they go because everyone else does. They really do not have any idea as to what they want to do or how they are going to do it. Their current job is just a filler. When something goes wrong or things get tough, chances are they will quit that job and try something else until that becomes an unbearable task, as well. People who go to work because they want to better themselves and who have a list of goals they want to accomplish are going to be successful and stick with it. They evaluate themselves based on their own performance and figure out what the next step needs to be. Failure is not an option for them. If something does not work, they know what to avoid the next time. Pretty soon they will have conquered their goal and will move on to the next one. If you compare these people to those who roll out of bed with no plan, you can see how some people never finish anything or get anywhere in life.

Age of Accomplishment

To many people, age is a very big deal. Some people do not want to tell others how old or young they are; they may lie about their age, and many get uncomfortable when they are asked how old they are. In today's society some believe that a person's worth is largely based on their age and that a person's age reflects the presence or lack of certain abilities. The reality of the situation is that the more mature a person is, the more experience that person should have and be able to share with others. In the business world, some believe that being young is an advantage. Younger individuals may be very bright and have a lot to offer, but they need to partner their young enthusiasm and intelligence with a dose of experience. You would think most people would agree with this statement, but some may have a different perspective. The company with a young face may communicate more energy and ambition than the company with a more dated look. It is what it is. With this in mind, how does one create a younger and more energetic appearance that appeals to today's society? The answer is simple: proper nutrition and exercise. Your age is meaningless; it is your physical appearance that tells a story. It is really tough to pinpoint the age of people who are in good shape and who present themselves well. Fitness is not just about looks; it is also about energy. If you have a strong will and give off a good and healthy energy, you can make a powerful impression.

Typically, a younger person is considered to be healthy by default. There are some who think that people in their twenties are still too young to suffer any major health issues (unless, of course, they were born with some). Concerns begin to arise about those who are in their thirties, forties, and fifties. This does not mean these people are unhealthy. In fact many people sixty and older are still very healthy and should not be alarmed by this statement. In general the people who have led fast and hard lifestyles should be more concerned. Fifty is still considered young. Think about the presidential election. Candidates need to be in good health. The stress that comes with being the leader of the country can be very intense. If the candidate is not in good health before the election, who is going to feel comfortable with that person running the country? You are going to want someone who has a lot of experience but also is healthy enough to handle the pressures of the job. A healthy leader is a strong leader.

Age should be considered more of a mind-set. Depending on the type of shape you are in, your workouts should follow suit. If you are an avid weight lifter who is in top physical condition, you can continue to train hard and adapt as needed. If you are a more mature person who has not touched a weight in years, you need to start slow and assess your tolerance level before you increase your workload. Understanding your personal limitations is very important when establishing a routine. However, what you believe to be your limitations should not be an excuse for how much you push yourself. If you look for an easy way out, you are only cheating yourself.

People over the age of forty may want to focus more on weight control and developing lean muscle mass. Unless you are a seasoned or professional weight lifter, you may want to avoid lifting very heavy weights and eating large amounts of food to increase muscle size and density. This is only a suggestion, as you know your body better than anyone else. If you believe you can still lift like a champion, go for it. Otherwise, it may be time to focus more on the long-term health benefits of exercising and eating the right foods. Too much of anything can turn into a negative. If you abuse your body with years of hard, heavy, improper, and careless weight lifting or play an extremely demanding physical sport, you risk feeling and looking just as bad as the people who partied all the time and never took care of themselves. Everything you do should be balanced according to your level of health and activity.

Consider retired athletes; many of those who played way past their prime were a mess. They spent their whole career pushing harder and training to be the best at their profession.

They did not know when to quit. It is a very admirable mind-set, but common sense needs to be applied. They may not have given much thought to their health when they retired. This does not apply to everyone, though. Today, through research and improved training protocols, trainers and athletes are better prepared for the long haul in their sport. The coaches' and the trainers' jobs are supposed to focus on preparing athletes for competition and getting the most out of them. In professional sports it is believed that the body can only peak for so long before things begin to slow down. Training for a sport is a healthy thing to do, but overtraining can be very dangerous. Those who do overtrain leave themselves wide open to getting injured and not being able to recover. Many professional athletes retire in their mid- to late thirties, which most people still consider to be pretty young. Taking the appropriate measures to stay in shape throughout the years is a very wise practice to get into.

When a person is no longer in his or her prime, it can be a hard thing to deal with. Not only does the body feel beat up, but the ego can take a huge hit, as well. Playing it smart and knowing when to back off can be life changers. You may laugh about the things you cannot do easily anymore until you cannot do them at all. It is scary and depressing to realize you are no longer capable of doing something you used to be good at. It can be a psychological trauma that can trigger a low morale. You may ask yourself how you would recover from something like that. In this case prevention is the best cure. Not training is bad, overtraining is bad, and not planning for your future is even worse. You do not need to have every minor detail ironed out but you should have an idea of how you want to end up. You may not have played a professional sport but will still face many of the same decisions when it comes to your health and fitness.

It is best to train intelligently. Training like an animal or not training at all will leave you in a place many do not want to be in. Everyone wants to win the race, but sometimes keeping pace behind the lead is the best way to win in the end. Creating a plan that offers balance, flexibility, longevity, and room for innovation and unexpected circumstances is the smart way to go. Just because you are beyond your so-called prime does not mean that you can never get back in shape. That is the furthest thing from the truth. You are only as healthy as your mentality. There is a psychological component to true health. If you believe you are done and your body is wrecked, you will find getting in shape to be an uphill battle. Even if you only have a small desire to get fit, that little flame of ambition can grow into a raging inferno of results driven by cause and possibility. You will literally write your own ticket.

Excuses are just the mind's way of tricking your ego into believing things that aren't true. When you are young, it is easy to think you will not be affected when you are older. When you are older and realize that that is not true, it is easy to say that you were young and didn't know any better. At what point does the phrase "I was young and dumb" not apply anymore? Whether you are twenty-five or sixty-three, you can still use that same excuse as long as it applies to a time period when you were younger. It's kind of funny but very true. When hiding behind an excuse becomes too embarrassing to handle, change will take place with quickness and precision. It is all for the better.

There are many resources available that have to do with health and fitness, many of which may be contradictory. This can be very confusing to a new learner. Be careful who you trust for advice about your heath. Having a variety of sources to choose from can be a good thing, but if you are too confused as to who you should listen to, do your research. Different things work for different people. If you were studying to improve your attitude and read a book on positive attitudes, would that one book help you change your life completely? It may, but chances are you will need to reinforce the ideas you heard in the first book. What if the same author came out with another book about positive attitudes? You would have to expand on what you learned and make the adjustments. It is like fine-tuning an instrument. Your body is the instrument, and in order for it to play at its optimal level, it needs to be adjusted and readjusted. This will ensure it stays in peak physical condition. Information is changing all the time, and advancements are made every day. New discoveries and technology will forever change the way the human race operates as a whole. Your health and fitness are no different. Studying new information told and retold by different sources is the best way to learn and make it sink in. You should definitely have a favorite source, but adding to your wealth of knowledge and resources is a smart practice.

If you are more mature in age, you will want to make sure you are exposing yourself to the best information possible. You may ask yourself if it is more difficult to lose weight and get into shape after age fifty. The answer is for you to decide on an individual basis; no one can answer it for you. Most likely, your truth will not be the same as everyone else's. This cannot be stressed enough. Much of your progress in maintaining a fitness program—and in life, for that matter—will come from within you and how you think. If this is not your current way of thinking about the world and its offerings, perhaps it should be. It is not always easy to get someone to change old habits that have been established over a lifetime. It may take a serious event, like a heart attack, to make people aware there really is an issue with their health and the way they are treating their body. Only you can control what happens to you in your life; no one else is responsible.

There may never be a perfect time to start something, but you can still start. You may know people who have spent their whole life coming up with excuses as to why they will start "tomorrow." They may cite such obstacles as work, family, sickness, being tired, not having enough money, an impending move, inclement weather, and so on. Does any of this sound familiar? If it does, then you should know what you have to do. Do not delay any further; start today. You cannot reach the top of the staircase by jumping but you will eventually reach it if you start by taking it one step at a time.

Your Time Is Important

Awareness is the power that is concealed within the present moment.... The ultimate purpose of human existence, which is to say, your purpose, is to bring that power into this world.

—ECKHART TOLLE

Your time here on Earth is special, and you should try to enjoy every waking moment as much as possible. When you first started out, time seemed to be so abundant. You assumed that whatever you could not get done that day could be handled another day. You may have thought that any time wasted and not used productively could be made up somewhere down the road. After all, time is on your side. Isn't it?

People often begin a task with so much excitement and energy but then do not finish what they start. They get caught up somewhere along the way, and all of their excitement seems to fizzle out. To a child, hopes and dreams are so real and attainable. A child's mind is so pure, free, and untouched that it is easy for them to be wishful and hopeful. Unlike adults, who have had some rough experiences and been walked on a few times, children are able to imagine and create a world where everything works out in their favor. What some believe to be merely a fantasy is reality to a young and uncorrupted mind. Children's dreams are alive and well, and most children have every intention of following through with them until they are a reality.

People learn that as they get older, the once-perfect perception they had of the world can be dashed away as easily as they can forget their own childhood. The happy and unburdened memories of being a child can quickly be replaced with what many believe to be the real truth. If you carry around this ugly and dark perception of the world, how can you protect yourself from becoming a victim? If you feel it is too late and you believe you are already a victim, how can you heal yourself and become happy again?

Here is your answer: it begins with you. You need to realize that you are in the driver's seat and control everything that happens in your life. You need to take responsibility for yourself and your actions. You cannot blame other people for what happens to you. You are ultimately responsible for whatever happens. Everything needs to be in your control if you are ever going to live a happy and successful life. If you make an excuse and tell yourself it is not your fault, you are really saying that you are not in control.

Snap Out of It

Life is all about energy. Energy is around you, part of you, and exchanged through you. Energy is a power that operates on a frequency. This power can gain momentum in one direction and then switch to run in another direction. How helpful this energy really is depends on what frequency you are operating on.

If you are headed down a negative path and are feeling negative energy, you need to snap out of it. Understand the power you have over your mind and body and use it to your advantage. Depending on how skilled you become at this, you may be able to change right away. Most people who have been operating on a negative frequency for a while need some time to adopt a more positive state of mind. For example, if a fan is spinning at a high speed and you pull the plug, the fan will still spin for a few moments. The fan had a lot of momentum before the plug was pulled and still has some residual energy left over. Eventually the fan will stop and be at rest. Your mind works that same way. You need to clear your mind of the old ideas that weren't working (similar to the fan spinning in the wrong direction) before you can replace them with something new. This period of clarification allows for a more successful transition into a new thought process.

It may take a little while for you to switch your thinking over to a more positive state of being. You can always try the quick route and change your outlook on a moment's notice, but for most people, it takes a little bit of time to make the adjustment. An example of this would be sticking something into the fan to make it stop right away. To make a permanent change, you need to be highly skilled at controlling and converting your energy levels at a moment's notice. These types of skills take some practice and getting used to. They involve training your mind to reach a higher level of enlightenment. It may take some time and patience, but anyone can do it with enough persistence. Everyone evolves at different rates. You will not know what level you are at until you try this for yourself.

You must realize that all of this wonderful time you thought you had is beginning to wane a tiny bit. As you get older, your life, which started out so simple and pure, begins to get bogged down with stuff to do. Whether you have a family to take care of or some major work commitments, you are a busy person who is only going to get busier. But it's OK, because you will have some time to do your stuff later on. Right now you need to get other people's stuff done for them. All the time you thought you had is now being spent on things you don't necessarily enjoy doing but must do. School is taking up your time, as are the studying and homework you must do. Pretty soon you have a job that is taking up more of your precious and abundant time. On top of that, you have a family to worry about. Maybe someone is sick and you need to take care of them or you have kids who need their lunch packed so you can get them off to school. Don't forget to walk the dog before you head off to work yourself. With all of these basic and normal daily activities that need attending to, what happened to your time? When do you get to sit down and focus on just you? Can you even focus on just yourself anymore? What is your plan to regain some of the time you have been spending on everyone but you?

Although you remember starting out with all the time in the world, you can't help but feel like there is not enough of it. Someone or something is consuming your energy and not leaving much for you. Maybe this describes you, and maybe it doesn't. Many people lead very busy lives with school, family, two jobs, and other circumstances that take up much of their free time. It is easy to get so caught up in what is expected of you and what everyone else is doing that you just simply forget to take care of your own needs. If you don't do it, who will? If you want something done right, do you need to do it yourself?

It does not have to be this way. With all of this chaos going on, you have forgotten to take care of the most important person—you. Your feelings and emotions will play a very important role in your ability to regain your sense of freedom, health, and spare time. How you perceive the world around you is exactly how it is, and no one or nothing can change that unless you want it to.

If you feel like your health could be better, it is time to take charge of your life again. You may not have any obvious problems at the moment but know you could be doing just a little bit better. That is a very smart and admirable admission. There are several reasons why it would be good for you to get in better shape.

The ideas shared and discussed in this book are going to help you put things into perspective—your perspective. How you want your life to be is how it is going to be when you take the proper steps. You are the ultimate controller of your time. The joy you experience in those waking moments is completely up to you. Use this book as an outline for your freedom. Your results will be evident as you put the principles in the following pages to use. Read and reread this book as many times as you deem necessary. Use it as a reference for building your dream body and reaching your ideal level of success. Congratulations on making up your mind to be a healthier you! May you find happiness and everlasting success.

The Haters Club

One person's jealousy is another person's triumph. It is in this jealousy that others are exposed to their own weaknesses.

—RYAN WEBER

This may be hard to believe, but not everyone is going to see your venture to ultimate fitness the same way you do. This is a journey talked about by many and completed by some. It would definitely be easier to get in shape working with a group of people, but even if you only find one partner, you will be way ahead of the rest. If you have to begin training by yourself, you are still better off than if you didn't do it at all. Encouragement from a family member or close friend can be a great boost of confidence. It would be exciting and motivating if your friends shared the same ambition to get in shape with you. However, if it doesn't happen this way, do not become discouraged. You can succeed and prove it to yourself on your own. Ultimately, you are responsible for your own failure or success. It's up to you to create the motivation that will inspire others to follow in your footsteps. Some may despise you for trying.

Everyone hears about hard work and dedication, but not everyone understands it or gets to see it. Being an advocate for the fitness lifestyle will help you understand it very well, since you will be living it day in and day out. Once you begin to see and feel the improvements you are making in your life and body, you will have a new appreciation for yourself. This is a wonderful feeling that will follow you everywhere you go. It will pour out of you like the sun warming the Earth on a summer's day. People will begin to notice a change in you and become curious about what it is you are doing. Some may compliment you, and some may not.

Those who do compliment you are secure with themselves and their lives. They understand discipline and are not afraid to commit and encourage others in their efforts. They are the ones who will ask you questions and want to share in the success you are achieving. They will be happy for you and want to be part of something good. To them, it's much wiser to lift people up than to pull people down. It would be in your best interest to make friends with as many of these people as you can find.

On the flip side, not everyone will comment on your new appearance, but don't be fooled—they are noticing. These people believe they are not as fortunate as you are. For some reason there is a force that is always working against their happiness. No matter what they do, they cannot seem to find peace within themselves. If they do say something, it may be a snippy, negative comment. Don't let this bother you. They are usually displeased with their own situation and have to take it out on others to make themselves feel better. It is a fact of life that everyone experiences some form of stress sooner or later. Everyone handles their emotions and issues in life differently. Following through with your fitness goals will be a test of your dedication that proves how committed you truly are.

A Short Story

Sean was a good-looking but skinny kid in high school. He was fortunate to have good friends and ended up dating some of the girls in his class. When he graduated and left for college, he became interested in working out. After seeing some photos of the current bodybuilding and fitness models, he decided to improve his own body and see how far he could take it.

In the meantime, Sean had begun dating an attractive girl from his class. She had a great personality and was a lot of fun. Unfortunately, it didn't work out for Sean and his girlfriend. They decided to go their separate ways and chase their dreams. He continued to work out and improve his body to the point where he started getting noticed by people. Most of his buddies didn't understand all that he did to stay in shape and why he did it. Nonetheless, after some light kidding around, they didn't judge him either way. They actually thought it was great that he was sticking with it.

Years later Sean was offered an opportunity to do some fitness modeling. Although he was still in shape, he definitely had some work to do if he was going to be in a photo shoot. He trained hard, ate right, and lost the weight to prepare for this special opportunity. The day came for Sean to do his photo shoot. After spending several hours working with the photographer, Sean had a small portfolio of pictures. It was a relatively small accomplishment but was a big deal for Sean.

Once he had lost some weight and made obvious improvements to his body, many of his friends grew curious and asked him what he was doing. Sean told his buddies that he was doing some fitness modeling and needed to get in shape for the pictures. His buddies thought it was a little much but still supported him. One day Sean ran into his old girlfriend at the store. She was excited to see him but asked what he had done to himself. She told Sean that he looked too thin and that no girls worth mentioning would ever be attracted to a guy who looked like him. She noticed his muscular physique and suggested he fatten up a little bit if he ever wanted to date a good-looking girl again.

She went on to give him several examples of what she thought a real man would look like. She told him that she wanted a man with some meat on his bones—love handles—and that walking around with extra fat was normal. According to her, only obsessive-compulsive people worked out to lose weight. She claimed that she gave up a chance at a modeling career because she didn't want to be known as "one of those crazy people." She also said she could eat whatever she wanted and remain beautiful and attractive to men. Her ideal man would be able to eat whatever he wanted, as well.

Sean's friend, though still very attractive, had put on some extra weight. It seemed that she was trying to make Sean feel bad so she would feel better about her current situation. Sean listened to her respectfully but knew that none of her advice was helpful or necessary. Sean was in great health and looked pretty good. This was not the case for his ex-girlfriend. Fortunately for Sean, he had a new girlfriend who was quite pretty herself. His current girlfriend appreciated the fact that he was in shape and shared his passion for being fit. When he told her about his experience with his ex, his current girlfriend laughed and told Sean, "She is only saying that because she knows she doesn't look as good as you do with her clothes off. She knows you look good naked and is probably a little insecure about how her body looks now." Sean wasn't looking for an opinion either way, but the recent events were no surprise to him. Miserable people like to keep company with other miserable people. If they see people who are happy, they are sometimes compelled to bring them down to their level. It's sad but very true.

You never know exactly what another person is thinking, but in the above case, it's safe to say that Sean's ex-girlfriend was either jealous of him or insecure about her own body. This example demonstrates some of the different views and opinions others may have of you and your success. You don't have to agree with any of them, let alone listen to any of them. It's up to you to ignore the negativity and move on with your progress. If you stop and listen to everyone who claims to have an idea that is better than yours, you would never have time to pursue any endeavors yourself. Continue to be yourself and let the haters worry about themselves.

There is no denying that your health is important and will affect the kind of life you live. You are not expected to drop weight and try out for a modeling competition, but if you work hard and the opportunity presents itself, take it. There are several reasons why others might not like you improving yourself. Do not be concerned with what these people have to say. Most likely there is something going on in their life that they are not happy with.

Sometimes their behavior is a form of manipulation and control. They may be jealous and feel like they have to bring you back down to their level or lower to make themselves feel good again. They can't accept the fact that you are improving your life because they don't share the same ambition and drive that you do. Though they will never admit it, your success can be intimidating to them. You are doing everything you are supposed to be doing, and it's working. Their negativity comes from something else; it's not anything you have done. You cannot change them, nor can anyone else. They have to realize what they are searching for on their own.

They may be spewing negativity in every direction, but they are the ones who are suffering the most. Motivational speaker Bob Proctor said, "Acid destroys the vessel in which it sits." Some people look for any reason to bring others down. If you have to, go out and make some new friends who accept you for who you are. There are definitely many other people out there who are supportive and will help to encourage you. If you stay positive, the right people will come into your life, brightening it up all the way.

Reframing

A man who is master of himself can end a sorrow as he can invent a pleasure. I don't want to be at the mercy of my emotions. I want to use them, to enjoy them, and to dominate them.

— OSCAR WILDE

The idea of reframing comes from the field of neurolinguistic programming (NLP). This technique was made popular by the self-help guru Anthony Robbins. The idea behind NLP is that your words help create your thoughts. Your thoughts are rooted deep in your nervous system, and subconsciously you are creating the mind frame of success or failure with your words. NLP is a form of self-programming in which your choice of vernacular influences your overall outcome and how you respond to different situations. When you understand this, you can use it to your advantage. You have the power to choose how you respond to people and situations.

For example, instead of giving in to someone's jealousy, you could reframe the idea as something more positive. Tell yourself that what you are hearing is good news, rather than bad news. An individual who recognizes your efforts enough to make a comment, even if it's negative, shows you that you are doing something right. You are on the right path, are doing the right things, and are being noticed. Disregard the person's negativity and congratulate yourself for reaching the next level. You are now in a desired position in life.

When you are around negative people, keep your thoughts to yourself. Don't try to convince the haters to see things your way, as they probably won't listen. They can't go where you are going and they aren't meant to. Be polite and excuse yourself from their presence and their negative nature. They have their own personal issues they are dealing with and only want to spread the misery. Their pain and suffering on the inside are showing on the outside. You should be able to laugh this off while thinking, "if it were easy, then everyone would be doing it." Maintain your own happiness and hold on to your feeling of accomplishment.

Love is the medicine that heals all. It is through your unwavering faith and love that good things come. Consider these words from Gautama Buddha: "Hate is not conquered by hate.

Hate is conquered by love. This law is eternal." The best way to handle negative people who cannot keep their opinions quiet is to simply love them. Let them know you hold no animosity toward them, despite their feelings of hate. You accept them for who they are and wish them the best in life. In time, these people will realize they are not getting through to you and leave you alone. They will either recognize they need to make a change themselves or they will focus their attention on someone else who pays them proper mind and attention. You can do all this while maintaining the proper balance and harmony you want for your own life.

In Chinese philosophy, the yin and yang are supposed to represent the idea of balance and harmony. This idea represents a type of freedom for those who embrace it. Those who understand love and balance live wonderful and peaceful lives. Philosophy may not be studied by everyone, but this example lends credence to the phrase "beauty is in the eye of the beholder." Should it be your eye that catches this philosophy, you can be the one who lives in peace and harmony.

Something Else to Keep in Mind

If everyone in the world had the same opinion, would the opinion be valuable? The fact that people are entitled to their own ideas and thoughts about a particular subject is great news. If everyone thought the same way, originality would not exist. This is a pretty obvious statement but is one that is often overlooked. You need to experience the bad so you can recognize and appreciate the good.

In Greek mythology, there is a story about Philoktetes. He was a Greek archer who, on his journey to do battle in the Trojan War, was bitten by a snake. The snake bit his ankle and caused a wound that became infected and began to bother the other sailors on the journey. The stench of the wound became so unbearable that the crew decided to abandon him on the island of Lemnos. They then continued on their journey. When they arrived and engaged in combat with the enemy, they did not fare well and asked the gods for guidance to help them win. They were told that they needed Philoktetes to win the war. His festering wound was full of the knowledge they needed to win the war.

The idea behind this story is that wounds can be helpful. Wounds are valuable and teach you lessons. They add to your originality and help you to stand out from the crowd. You can learn so much more through a loss or a failure than you can by having everything go your way. People grow through enduring pain. This can help you build a tremendous amount of character. It can help you appreciate the good and the bad life has to offer. Look at wounds not as an impossible obstacle but rather as opportunities for something better to come about.

6

It's All Business

Nobody talks about entrepreneurship as survival, but that's exactly what it is and what nurtures creative thinking.

— A N I T A   R O D D I C K

You and the Interview

If you asked your friends and family why they go to work, you would probably expect the answer may be to say that they work to earn a living. Some people go to college to receive a higher education, and others decide to start working straight out of high school. Whether you flip burgers for a living or are a high-level executive, how well you do your job directly affects somebody's livelihood and business. How you conduct yourself on a daily basis speaks volumes to a potential employer. The more you educate yourself and show initiative, the better your chances are of being presented with greater opportunities in the workplace. Careers are not just given to people; they are built and earned with respect and hard work. There may be some people who can skate through life with little drive and ambition and still do all right for themselves. But most people must compete in an overpopulated pool of hopeful and competent employees who are looking for a good solid career, just as you are (unless, of course, you are able to establish yourself as a leader and create your own success through investments, operating your own business, or becoming an entrepreneur).

In today's economy the job market is saturated with an abundance of people looking for work. The employers hold all of the power as to who they will select for a particular job and can truly have their pick of the mill. The competition is fierce! You may be the most qualified person for the position you are applying for, but how can you make yourself stand out from the others? Many people can fill out the application and list their qualifications and accomplishments while showcasing their enthusiasm and abilities. Once you get the interview, you have a chance to impress your prospective employer with your résumé, experience, and communication skills, but there is something else that can add to your chances of getting hired.

There is another personal attribute that can set you apart from the rest of the competition.

Being able to master the interviewing process is an important skill that requires practice. It's no secret that certain people interview better than others, but it is more than just being a good interviewee. There are many determining factors that can separate one person from the next. Education, communication skills, experience, and the way you present yourself are all important to an employer. It is up to you to make yourself stand out from the rest. What will set you apart from the crowd are your physical appearance and confidence. Everyone possesses a certain type of pizzazz. You may not be applying for a sales position, but your ability to sell yourself is very important.

When your prospective employer first lays eyes on you, he or she will subconsciously make an assumption about what kind of person you are. People always have and always will label and categorize others according to their appearance and likability. Your physical appearance can be a combination of many things; your level of confidence, the way you dress, how you speak, your level of energy, and your presence when you walk into a room are all fair indicators of your character. Your level of fitness has a direct impact on all of these traits. The shape of your body and your level of attractiveness are most likely the first things someone is going to notice about you and judge you on. Although you may disagree and feel uncomfortable with the idea, you probably do the same thing to others the first time you meet them. It is human nature, and on a subconscious level, everyone does it. This doesn't mean that if you are not good-looking and in shape, you won't ever get a job, but it does reveal how you can gain a competitive edge over someone else. This is a power that is completely in your control to develop and put into action.

This theory of likability parallels the idea of mate selection very closely. For example, when you select a significant other, you are going to be attracted to the other person for some reason or another. You may not be able to pinpoint what it is about the other person but you have a good or bad feeling about the person right away. Attraction isn't a choice, whether you like it or not. You have no control over your instinctual feelings about another person, just like you have no control over your first impression of another human being. However, you do have the ability to practice methods of improving your own likability, physical fitness, and appearance. You do not have to be an Adonis to secure the job that you want but you should at least be in shape and make a strong first impression. Physical fitness should be an important attribute that you productively work on improving while you apply and interview for an important position with a prospective employer.

In many fields, there are more people looking for work than there are jobs available. Considering the high unemployment rates, you can be sure the competition is much greater. Regardless of what people may think or tell you about first impressions, once an impression is made of you, it can be hard to change it, especially if it is made in a short period of time, such as during an interview. The window of opportunity to establish yourself as a viable candidate is small, and you need to make it count. Your physical appearance is the first impression an employer will have about the type of worker you are. Getting in shape will definitely give you more confidence and will convey to the employer that you care enough to invest in yourself and that that is how you are going to treat his company should he extend you the offer. If you do not believe this, you should go out and experiment for yourself. Look around at the people who are getting the jobs these days. Just be careful you do not blow any opportunities you may regret. It could cost you big time.

This can be viewed as unfair, but the reality of the situation is that it happens, probably more than anyone would ever like to admit. It's very reasonable to assume you may get the job over those who don't present themselves as well as you do. There are trained professionals who organize whole workshops based on first impressions and appearance. Everything from grooming, to personal hygiene, to the type of clothes you wear, to physical appearance is considered a target area to master before the interview. After all, you will be representing somebody's company. If it were your company, how would you want your employee representing you? Most likely, you would want the most competent and well-put-together person you could find. Your physically fit appearance will cause others to assume you have it together. Think about the presidential election. The majority of past presidents were individuals who were healthy and presented themselves well. Candidates have lost favor with the American people because of health issues and concerns. No one wants to elect a person who may not be healthy enough to complete the term. Being president is a very large responsibility and is highly stressful. Those who do get elected into office age significantly faster, even if they are in shape.

On the other hand, if a company is looking to downsize to a smaller number of employees, a physically unfit individual who is struggling at work may be on the chopping block. This is not to say that looks are everything, but a successful company has an image to maintain. That image is not just based on the company's reputation of doing business; it's also represented by the employees themselves. An employee who is driven and takes initiative most likely keeps in shape. A physically fit employee is also most likely going to cost less in insurance. Have you heard about some companies not hiring smokers? According to the *New York Times*, people who smoke miss an average of average of 7.67 more days per year compared to non-smokers. Why do you think that is? The negative affects of cigarette smoke include, but are not limited to headache, insomnia, heart disease, and mental depression. Motivated people don't make excuses. If there is an obstacle in front of them, they confront it head on and find a way around it. These are the kind of people a company will be sure to try to keep around. If you keep in shape but are bigger than the guy who was skinny all his life, do not feel you should worry about your job or image. Fitness is just as much attitude as it is looks. Your employer will know the difference between a go-getter and a skater. You can be sure of it.

If you work in an office and have to sit at a desk all day, a few pounds of weight gain is understandable, but this is not a green light to allow yourself to become obese and ignore your physical health and appearance. Drinking soda and eating cheese puffs is not a good way to occupy your time while sitting at the computer and fielding phone calls. You should definitely be paying attention to what you eat and drink throughout the day. It doesn't look good to your employer if you allow yourself to become sloppy and out of shape. What you are really saying is that your work ethic isn't as strong as your employer previously thought. It can also be disrespectful to your coworkers, depending on how out of hand it gets. This may be a harsh reality, but people are talking, whether you think they are or not. Have some self-respect and be successful in your career by staying fit. Prove to your employer you are still the hardworking and diligent hire that you were when you first began.

The workplace is a tough environment to stand out in, as there is always a lot of competition going on. Make sure you stay on top of your game. If you are up for a promotion or you are looking for a new job, remember that to be a desirable candidate, you should:

1. Take pride in your appearance and style of dress
2. Take good physical care of yourself
3. Practice exercise and good nutrition daily
4. Become an avid goal setter
5. Invest in yourself and strive to improve on a daily basis

6. Become a team player if you are not already
7. Practice being high energy and taking initiative
8. Take all criticism as constructive

There is much to be desired in the workplace. Use the idea of fitness as a catalyst to improve yourself and be a better you. Let your coworkers notice for themselves the positive changes that will be taking place when you take control of your health and image. Do not get caught up in trying to change things that are out of your control. Appreciate the fact that you have recognized an opportunity to stand out and be different from everyone else. Employers, customers, and coworkers alike will all notice your drive and determination without you having to bring it to their attention. The more confidence you have, the less you will feel you need to talk about it. When it comes to your fitness, being informed and prepared is better than being pessimistic and in denial. Take the time to improve your physique and do not let laziness or a negative attitude get the best of you.

The Mr. Moon Story

A large gentleman who goes by the name Mr. Moon is a guidance counselor for high school kids. He is roughly six feet five inches tall and 260 pounds of muscle, not fat. He looks like he should be playing football for the Philadelphia Eagles, rather than working in a school. He is well liked by the staff and faculty at the school and has a great rapport with the students. With a level head and calm demeanor, he manages to be very firm and serious in his advice to the students. When speaking with him, most people get the feeling that he genuinely cares and believes in the good he is doing. The kids look up to and respect Mr. Moon. He has class and has a style all his own that resonates with authority and makes a solid statement. Anyone who meets him in person and shakes his hand knows right away that he is a force who chooses to be gentle, rather than domineering.

High school kids are not always the most respectful. Maybe they didn't pay attention to the values and discipline taught at home, or maybe they were never taught any manners. Poor attitudes can develop from a lack of something or disgust. Many adults feel it necessary to express their concern about the lack of respect kids have these days. If you were to turn on the news and see a report of a high school student beating up his teacher or coach, you probably would not be that surprised anymore. It is still disturbing but it happens. Thankfully, the majority of society can still function on a respectful level. But some people can't, and this brings to light a more serious concern about how to ensure that these kids will listen to and respect authority.

What do you do when a student starts to get verbally disrespectful with the teachers? Unruly teenagers can be rebellious and do not consider the consequences of their actions. The threat of an English or math teacher to send a student to detention does not have the same effect as it once did. The use of paddles and rulers for temper control is now frowned upon by society. The student will stand up to the teacher and say "I don't care" and mean it. Things can escalate rather quickly, and at that point, something more must be done. A five-foot-tall and 120-pound English teacher most likely will not intimidate a misguided and adolescent youth. Instead of arguing with the student and waiting for something more to happen, the teacher sends the individual down to have a visit with Mr. Moon.

Imagine the following scenario for a moment. A student who is five feet ten inches tall and weighs 150 pounds is told to go talk to Mr. Moon. The physical threat the students encounter when they visit him is relatively large. What is the likelihood that they will get verbally abusive with this guy? Even if they were having a really bad day and did want to assault Mr. Moon, would they really stand a chance? Probably not, as they would be too worried about how bad they would get tuned up if they actually did say something wrong or threatened any kind of disobedience. Not only are they aware of his dominance, but they also respect him as a person. When students are instructed to see Mr. Moon, they have to explain to him what they did to get sent down for the visit. This is most likely awkward and uncomfortable for the students, who are already sold on the idea of what can happen if they mess up in the presence of Mr. Moon. In return, Mr. Moon treats the students fairly and listens to what they have to say. He could just stand there and yell at them about how they should not have messed up in the first place, but he takes a different approach. His dominant presence and his respectful treatment of the students are a recipe for success.

Mr. Moon is a genuinely nice guy and does very well with the students. He listens to what they have to say before he speaks. He is respectful of the students and treats them the way he wants to be treated. He talks to them like they are adults and gives them real advice that could make a difference in their lives. The students seem to respond well to what he has to say. However, you can bet that if a student does becomes lippy and disrespectful to Mr. Moon, the possibility of what can happen is much scarier than a written detention. Hands that can palm a basketball can also fit around the skull of a teenager. The students choose to listen to Mr. Moon. His physically dominating presence and respectful manner are a powerful combination that works. If he were a domineering bully, he might not get through to the kids. Putting a soft edge around a huge threat is a very effective tactic when it comes to delicate dealings and interactions. Everyone who understands fitness and the alpha male can also appreciate being treated fairly. Striking a balance between the two is a good practice to get into. If you do not possess the qualities yourself, you can start to develop them.

This is a great example of what physical dominance can help you accomplish in the real world. You can probably remember a time when you met someone and thought to yourself, "I sure am glad he is on my side." An individual's physical prowess is clearly an indicator of the potential the individual may have. When used for good, fitness is an excellent tool to develop for leverage in your personal life. This is a trait that can successfully be applied in teaching, coaching, and business. A great teacher knows that a little bit of fear is an aid in developing a disciplined student. A student will then respect the power that his superior possesses. Physical fitness is a tool you can take with you no matter what you decide you want to be in life.

Creating an Advantage

You can get much further with a kind word and a gun than you can with a kind word alone.

— A L   C A P O N E

In business, people are always looking for the edge to make themselves more competitive in the marketplace. A successful businessman has too many qualities and strategies to list, but suffice it to say that appearance and presence can make a big difference in the type of image you portray. The old saying "dress for success" proves to be important in the business world. While being physically attractive can earn you a few points, an even better quality to possess that commands attention from everyone is a fit and toned physique. In order to be successful and on top of your game, you want to have a strong physical presence and good body language. A UCLA professor named Albert Mehrabian, completed research in 1967 demonstrating that words account for only 7 percent of your communication; the other 93 percent is conveyed through your tone of voice and body language. It is interesting to note that your body language communicates much more than the actual words themselves. With this in mind, how much of an impact do you think your physical appearance is going to have on your next sales transaction?

There is something to be said about people who take care of themselves. Everyone notices the person who walks into the room and is built and in shape. Whether you are a man admiring the slim waist and curves of a woman or a woman appreciating the big arms and chest on a man, you are noticing something. When combined with a pleasant and respectful attitude, being fit portrays a level of confidence that many people will admire. You can't help but feel good about that kind of person, unless you are the out-of-shape and jealous type yourself. If you do resent this type of a person, you may have a problem.

You can bet the people who are in shape are willing and able to keep up with the fast pace of sales. It takes a high-energy, motivated, and fit individual to stay ahead of the competition. The healthier you are, the more stamina you have, which will enable you to be more productive. Higher productivity equals more money and a happier customer base. Businesses rely heavily on their sales staff and need them to be successful. The top companies want the best sales staff and will pay more to get it. Fitness is your secret weapon. Although practiced by few, it is attainable by all.

Positioning

There are a number of different skill sets that are needed in order to become a success. No one knows how talented you are just by looking at you, but everyone can respect an individual who projects a strong sense of vitality and well-being. Your presence is directly correlated with your physical appearance. The individual who has it together is going to stand out like a giraffe in a herd of elephants. There are so many subtle things that the subconscious mind picks up on. For example, you know you have a business meeting at 9:00 a.m. You set your alarm for 6:00 a.m. and lay out all of your clothes and everything you will need for the day. After your morning cup of coffee and breakfast bar, you are off to the gym. You spend an hour completing an awesome cardio and weight-lifting session. You shower, get dressed, and eat the healthy breakfast you packed for yourself the night before. On your drive to the morning meeting, you feel refreshed and energized. That excitement and enthusiasm spills over into your presentation, and you perform at your personal best. Your energy, physical presence, and attitude about life in general speak volumes. You are prepared, and people can tell you are ambitious and motivated. Right away this communicates something different about you and makes you more marketable. You are able to separate yourself from the crowd and convey a certain level of competence. You are able to build upon your functionality as a professional and conduct yourself with a strong drive to achieve your goals. Your elevated status is going to distinguish you from others in the room. This is all just a side effect of practicing a healthy and fit lifestyle.

When you wake up and look in the mirror to dress for work, remember that your appearance will affect your whole demeanor. Being in shape and looking good will make you feel good. You will have more energy when you go out in the world and have interactions. The more positive you are, the better chance you will have of being met with the same in return. When you talk to your customers with a more positive attitude, you will attract more business. More business will equal more money and will lead to opportunities you may not have had if you weren't mentally prepared and confident. You also will be equipped with the energy to stay aggressive and competitive.

Fitness is a single component you can use to help build upon and better your professional life. Being fit and physically dominant will give you more confidence and the ability to grab the attention and respect of those around you. However, you need to be careful not to be too dominant. If you rely too much on your physical makeup and forget to maintain a reasonable and professional attitude, you may come across as domineering. As a result, your peers will think you are a jerk and will not want to do business with you. There is a big difference between being a dominant person and being a domineering person. You do not want to be classified as one of those brainless meatheads who stick their chest out a little too far. Whether people are afraid of you or not, there is always someone bigger and bad-der. Push a little too hard, and your coworkers will be happy to make the introduction for you. Although you may be able to inflate your ego, your personal and business life will suffer. There should always be a balance between brains and brawn.

Physical fitness is a gift that will serve you everywhere you go. People respect muscle and will want to stay on your good side for fear of what could happen if they don't. This idea of fear may sound kind of funny, but it is true. There are not too many big people who get picked on, unless they are large and out of shape. Even then, people make sure they make their comments out of earshot of the person they are talking about. There is nothing like a large muscular individual who can smile and be polite with his associates. Someone who has the power to boss people around but chooses to be kind and helpful is the type of person everyone wants to be friends with. People like this are charming, and others like being around them. It is a comfortable and secure position to be in. This trait makes them one of the most likable people in the business. Positive, confident, and motivated people usually have the first shot at success.

Sabotage

Your physical fitness doesn't just give you an edge, it also helps to protect you. Whether in the workplace or on the street, size does matter. Think of a time when a coworker was not so honest. It might not have been personal against anyone, but at some point a peer may have cheated or lied to get ahead. No one has to know about it for it to have happened. People are out for themselves and will do what they can to make a buck, as long as they feel they can get away with it. Someone's position could be sabotaged without that person ever knowing the truth about what happened.

You can be pretty sure your coworkers will think twice about doing this to you if you are in good shape. You may never find out who tried to throw you under the bus, but what if you did? The whole office knows you are a pretty tough individual who keeps in shape. If you were to catch the person, you could do a whole lot of physical damage. Of course, you wouldn't do anything at the workplace, as you might lose your job. You're smarter than that, and everyone knows it. When you do leave work, however, you can confront the liar without anyone else knowing about it. Make sure it is just the two of you, with no one there to step in and help out the other guy. This is not an invitation to exercise brute force in the workplace but should illustrate the point that you are not the one to cross.

If someone has an ill thought toward you, most likely that person will weigh the consequences of any possible actions before doing anything. For example, think about the nerd in your workplace. People might view him as a weak and easy target who probably won't fight back. Well, what if the nerd used to play football back in the day and is 205 pounds of solid muscle? Do you really think people are going to screw with him just to find out? Probably not.

Body Language

Business professionals should understand that body language is a critical aspect of communication. Words are important, but your body is the instrument that conveys most of your message. Your physical appearance may be more important than you thought. If you are speaking with a client and are slumped over in your chair with a potbelly stretching your shirt, the client may not take you too seriously. The guy who is clean-cut, in shape, and looks like he takes care of himself is much more likely to get the business over the sloppy guy. Here are just a few of the reasons why:

- Sloppiness is not professional—ever!
- Physical fitness demonstrates that you don't just sit around on your downtime.
- If you don't waste time, you must be a good worker.
- If you are a good worker, you will most likely do the job well and complete tasks on time.
- A job well done will earn you repeat business and more income.
- People like a professional and clean appearance.

Even if you do not agree with the above statements, they are what people are thinking. Fitness equals money and demonstrates stability and integrity. Just because you are in shape doesn't mean that you have a free pass and cannot do any wrong. You still need to be a competent worker and honor the agreement. Fitness is simply one more tool you can use to help get your foot in the door and bust the piggy bank wide open. Don't waste time on the couch doing twelve-ounce curls and supplementing with junk food. Prepare the right way and train for your success. If you don't, the competition will.

If you are sitting down while reading this, sit up straight and put your shoulders back right now. Notice how it's easier to breathe and you feel more awake. When you are at your next meeting, keep this same posture and look your associates in the eye with confidence, knowing you possess the secret to stay ahead of your competitors. During your next phone conversation at work, adopt the same posture to boost your level of confidence and focus. Your energy levels should noticeably improve. Once you fine-tune this part of your professional career, others will respect the fact that you have a certain position of power that elevates you above the competition. But knowing is only half the battle; putting it into action is what will earn you the victory.

7
Introduction to Nutrition

Those who have no time for healthy eating will sooner or later have to find time for illness.

— EDWARD STANLEY

When it comes to fitness, nutrition is king. What you put in your body directly affects your energy levels and how you feel. If you don't supply your body with the fuel it needs to stay healthy, you're going to have a very difficult time achieving your fitness goals. Nutrition goes hand in hand with fitness and the way you look. Think of it like this: you own a very rare and exotic car that no one else in the world has. You take very good care of this car by keeping it clean, taking it to the mechanic for maintenance, and driving conservatively. You pay close attention to the roads for any hazards and conditions you should avoid. When you fill the car up with fuel, you don't just use regular, you use the premium. In fact, you were even given special instructions to use a certain kind of premium fuel for maximum performance. As long as you do this, your car will run great and be issue free. If you don't use the proper fuel, your car will still be able to run but the engine will not operate at its fullest capacity. In fact, you are setting up the potential for many future problems.

With this example in mind, think about your body. Your body is this very rare vehicle that no one else on the planet can duplicate. If you mistreat your body and feed it garbage, it's not going to be able to perform as it should. Even just using the average fuel doesn't guarantee optimal performance. If your body is not performing as it should, making improvements should be at the top of your goal list. Make wise choices when it comes to food and pick out the best possible choices available. To figure out what works best, you may have to experiment until you find a meal plan that fits.

The old saying "you are what you eat" is very true on many levels. You should not expect to eat greasy fries and hamburgers, wash it down with a liter of cola, and look like Brad Pitt in the movie *Fight Club*. Likewise, a fitness model preparing for a runway show does not eat a box of Twinkies or oatmeal cream pies before slipping into her dress. People who need to keep their bodies and skin tones in top shape understand this very well. Poor decisions lead to poor results, which can cost some people their career. This may be a bit extreme but clearly illustrates the impact food can have on you and your well-being.

Food is very addicting. For some this is bad news, but for you this is great news. Did you know that you can train your taste buds? This means that if you are used to eating unhealthy food, you have the opportunity to retrain yourself. Think about a piece of candy for a moment and ask yourself what it is about that candy that you like so much. The candy you are thinking of is most likely very sweet, though some may prefer salty and/ or sour candy. Now think about the habit of smoking cigarettes for a moment. When smokers light up and take the first hit of a cigarette, they are triggering a chemical reaction in their brains and bodies. This reaction gives them a sort of high, which they attribute to the cigarette. It is very well-known that the drug nicotine in a cigarette is addictive over a period of time. So how can a person who just started smoking claim to be addicted? Studies have shown that while some drugs have very high addictive tendencies from first contact, nicotine is not one of them. An individual would need to smoke several cigarettes over a prolonged period of time before actually becoming addicted.

Now back to that piece of candy. Just like with the cigarette example, people who eat a lot of candy can develop a type of addiction over time. Eventually if these people were to not get their sugar fix, they might actually get a headache and become agitated. This is the body's way of saying it wants that candy. So what can you do?

Rather than giving in and eating the candy, you can tell yourself no. This sounds pretty easy to do, but for some it can be very difficult. This gives you an opportunity to practice willpower. You need to make a choice about what you really want. You don't have to eliminate the candy completely from your diet, but you should begin to reduce the amount of it you consume. Just because you want to make healthier choices about the food you eat doesn't mean that you have to torture yourself and cut out everything you like. The key is to start making adjustments. For example, you can substitute an apple, grapes, or raisins for that piece of candy and still get your sugar fix. Over time, you will begin to crave apples, grapes, and raisins. You will be retraining your body to want healthier foods. Once you see how this is possible, it will be much easier for you to make the transition from unhealthy to healthy. Your body will expect and look forward to eating much better. This should definitely give you a big boost of faith and confidence.

One of the most important things you can do for yourself to make this process of being healthy a whole lot easier is to plan for it. When you know what your schedule looks like during the week, you can be prepared and make sure you eat healthy. Take a few minutes on Sunday morning to make a list of all the food and supplements you think you will need for the week. When you go out later in the day, you can pick up whatever you need from the store. That evening, depending on how busy your week is, you can cook your meals for the week ahead of time. Preparing meals is a great way to plan if you are short on time. Simply make a menu for the week, cook everything you will need, and freeze the meals until you are ready to eat them. This will save you a lot of time and ensure that you eat healthy meals throughout the week.

Generally speaking, nutritional needs vary and depend on the individual. Ethnicity, race, gender, and physical fitness all play a role in determining what your proper caloric intake should consist of. It is strongly recommended that before starting any kind of a diet or exercise regimen, you consult an experienced doctor and health-care practitioner.

When you sit down to eat a meal, how do you categorize the food you are about to eat? Food is fuel for your body and provides you with energy to accomplish all of your fitness goals.

It's not just a meal to fill you up until you are hungry again. Your meals should be well thought out and balanced to meet your individual needs. Everyone's needs are different, but the guidelines are the same. Each meal should consist of a healthy serving of protein, carbohydrates, fats, and fiber. Vitamins, minerals, and antioxidants also play key roles in keeping your body running at its optimal rate. So what do these nutrients mean to you?

Carbohydrates

Carbohydrates are the body's main source of energy. They can be divided into two main groups: simple sugars and complex carbs. Simple sugars are used up by the body at a rapid rate. These sugars are best eaten before and after a workout, since they will give you a quick burst of energy. They are used up and digested quickly for energy. Fruit, juice, honey, and raw sugar are examples of simple sugars.

Complex carbs are best when eaten as part of your regular meals. Complex carbs break down at a slower pace, keeping your energy at a more consistent level. Rice, pasta, potatoes, and oatmeal are good examples. You should always try to select these from a whole wheat or whole grain source. The difference between wheat and white breads and starches is that white breads are digested by the body at a faster rate and are not as good for you as whole grains, which are digested at a slower rate. Excess sugars that are not digested and used by the body are stored as fat, which can cause unnecessary weight gain. Whole grain food sources help to limit this problem because they are easier for the body to utilize and burn off.

Carbohydrates are classified by the glycemic index, which categorizes the rate at which each unit is used and digested by the body. The glycemic index is based on the amount of sugar contained in each food. The higher the amount of sugar they contain, the more you want to try to avoid them. The lower the amount of sugar they contain, the better they are for you. Carbs that are lower in sugar are digested at a more even rate, which is why they are recommended for your regular meals. There is less of a chance that these carbs will be stored as fat.

Insulin is important to mention at this point. Insulin is a hormone produced by the body that helps in regulating carbohydrate and fat metabolism. When you eat large amounts of carbs, your insulin levels spike and act to prevent your blood sugar from staying too high. All of the excess carbs that your body cannot use at the time are stored for future use. This means that rather than being burned up by the body's metabolism and used for energy, they are stored as fat. This is the main reason why you need to watch your carbohydrate intake, whether simple or complex. The time of day at which you consume either type of carb is also very important.

Proteins

Protein is the body's next source of energy. It is essential to cell growth and recovery and to building lean muscle mass. Without protein, there is no way for your body to repair itself and function properly. Protein should make up approximately 30 percent of your caloric intake, though this amount can vary depending on each person's level of physical activity and muscle mass. Typically a more active person is going to need to consume more protein, carbs, and fat.

There are two different categories of protein: complete and incomplete. Protein is made up of several different amino acids. A complete protein contains all of these amino acids. An incomplete protein lacks several of the amino acids, making it not as useful in building and repairing the body's cells and tissue. Remember to think in terms of balance. You want to make sure your food sources are as complete as possible to ensure you are meeting your requirements. If not, you will lack the nutrition needed to accomplish your fitness goals.

Good and complete sources of protein include red meat, chicken, fish, and dairy products. Supplementing with a protein shake is also an option if these foods are not readily available to you. A few examples of incomplete proteins are pasta, rice, beans, and bread. Many other foods do contain protein but not in the complete form you should be consuming. However, you can combine different sources together to make a complete form of this nutrient.

Fats

The third nutrient that needs to be included in your daily regimen is fat. Many people believe that fat is unhealthy and should be avoided as much as possible. Fat is a very necessary nutrient that is involved in several bodily functions. However, you do want to be careful how much you take in on a daily basis. Getting too much can cause several different health problems and stress your body. Meanwhile, not taking in any fat can be harmful, as well.

There are good fats and bad fats. Healthy fats promote cardiovascular health, hormone regulation, and neuromuscular function. Fat is measured in the body in the form of lipids and triglycerides. Cholesterol for example, is divided into two categories: high-density lipoproteins (HDL) and low-density lipoproteins (LDL). A healthy individual would expect to have a higher HDL (the good kind) than LDL (the bad kind). A simple blood test at your doctor's office will tell you what you need

to know. To have an accurate blood panel done, you must fast
for nine to twelve hours. This is to prevent any kind of a false
result, as certain nutrients can still be circulating in the bloodstream and would throw off the accuracy of the test.

With this general overview of nutrition, you now have a
better understanding as to why you need to eat healthier foods.
Eating well does not have to be a tortuous venture. You most
definitely can still enjoy your favorite foods, but you need to
make smart decisions. Depending on what your current fitness
level is and what you want it to be, your nutritional regimen
can be more intense or stay at an intermediate level. If you are
a beginner, the best way for you to start is to just jump in and
begin your program.

It is very is easy to make excuses as to why you should wait
to start your program. Whether it's your family or your business, you will always be able to find an obstacle in your way. The
difference between those who just say they will do something
and those who actually do it is huge. Talkers can stay talkers, but
walkers become joggers, who become runners, who end up
sprinting so hard toward the finish line that only positive results
and happiness can come their way. This is the part where you
get to feel really good about yourself for being a doer.

We were all given the same mind, body, and chance to succeed when we first started out. What you did with yourself
between then and now reflects the images and thoughts that
have been programmed in your mind. The good news is that
you have the power to make a choice. You have enough willpower and determination to influence hundreds, thousands,
and maybe even millions of people with your success story.
Your transformation began when you purchased this book and
will continue until you can write your own testimonial. Your
story will touch enormous amounts of people who want to be
just like you and take control of their lives. It all begins with
one thought. Your success can now become a reality.

Time to Get Inspired

Nike said it best with the slogan "Just Do It." Aside from being a very short and brilliant marketing campaign, it is very true. You need to jump right in to being healthy and learn as you go. There will be plenty of time to make adjustments and learn from mistakes. Mistakes are normal, and most people go through many of the same frustrations. If you have any doubts, just ask. There is plenty of support available to any fitness enthusiast who is looking for an edge. Those who offer nothing positive to say are just jealous that they don't possess the same amount of drive and integrity that you do. Be a doer and challenge yourself to reach new heights in your personal development.

Making an appointment with your doctor is always a good idea before you make any big changes in your lifestyle. Fitness is indeed a lifestyle. It's one that is both rewarding and challenging. You will see yourself grow physically, mentally, and socially and will make changes that are life altering. Not only will you look and feel better, but other people will notice you and respond to you differently. It is a tremendous feeling to have others compliment you on your progress.

It is important to give yourself a psychological advantage. For example, find a picture of the kind of look you are going for and would like to portray. Print it off the internet or cut it out of a magazine and put it in a place where you will see it often. This will help you to consistently visualize your goal. Want to go a step further? To add the ultimate advantage, take a picture of yourself and cut out your face. Now place the image of your face on the example picture you picked out for yourself earlier. This is equivalent to shifting your goal into overdrive. By creating an end result picture of yourself, you'll be able to more completely visualize what you are going to look like. If this sounds strange, just keep with it a moment. Every time you stare at that picture, you'll begin to build a new image of yourself. It's like looking in the mirror. Subconsciously, you can never move past the image you hold of yourself in your mind. Before you can change what's on the outside, you need to change and control what's on the inside. When you see yourself as a winner, you'll start to win.

Do not waste your time and energy creating reasons why you can't get into shape. The only thing standing in your way of producing positive results is limited thinking. Rather than thinking of ways to fail, create ways to accomplish. Wherever there is a problem, there is an opportunity for a solution. There is an upside to any downfall or low point. It may take a little searching and time on your part, but it's there for the taking. Instead of feeling sorry for yourself, use this knowledge to your advantage and retrain your mind to ask how.

How to Read a Nutrition Label

Before you can learn how to shop the right way, you will need to understand how to interpret what the food labels are telling you. Some are straightforward in telling you what is in the product, but others are not as clear. Knowledge is power. There is a lot of clever marketing that can go into a nutrition label, and sometimes it can be confusing.

In general, the nutrition facts on food labels are broken down as follows: Total fat includes saturated, trans, polyunsaturated, and monounsaturated fat. Next are cholesterol, sodium, and potassium. Carbohydrates are broken down into dietary fiber and sugars. Some labels will include soluble and insoluble fiber. Toward the bottom of the label, the amount of protein is listed. The vitamins and minerals are listed last. Depending on what you are buying, there may also be an ingredients list that will look similar to this:

Fats

Total fat is the first item listed on food labels. Your fat intake should be kept low, unless your doctor or nutritionist says otherwise. You especially want to stay away from saturated and trans fats, because they are more difficult for the body to break down. Trans fat is a processed fat and is the worst kind you can ingest. Unsaturated fats are more desirable. Your body does need a certain amount of fat to survive. While you want to keep it low, do not completely eliminate fats from your diet.

Cholesterol

Cholesterol is a type of fat that is made by the body and is also found in food. Your body does need some cholesterol, but too much is a bad thing. Cholesterol levels can be checked by a blood test. When your cholesterol levels are too high, a thick waxy deposit known as plaque can accumulate in your bloodstream, increasing your risk for heart attack and stroke. You should keep your dietary intake of cholesterol to a minimum.

Sodium

Sodium is a mineral and electrolyte used by the body to help regulate bodily functions. Sodium is also an important electrolyte used by the heart. Sodium occurs naturally in foods and is used as an ingredient in cooking. High levels of sodium can be harmful to you by increasing your risk of high blood pressure, stroke, and heart disease. You should try to keep your intake to around two thousand milligrams and should not exceed four thousand milligrams a day. A good habit would be to select low-sodium foods and minimize its use in cooking as much as possible.

Potassium

Potassium is a mineral and electrolyte that helps to keep the heart and many other organs in the body functioning properly. Low levels of potassium can lead to high blood pressure, digestive issues, and other diseases in the body. The recommended amount of potassium for a healthy individual is about 4,700 milligrams per day. Depending on your current diet, you may not be getting enough of this mineral.

Carbohydrates

Carbohydrates are one of the most widely talked about dietary nutrients. There is much debate as to what is the proper amount to take in on a daily basis. Even more important is what kind of carb you are ingesting. Carbs are the body's main source of energy and therefore are important. Depending on your nutritional goals, between one and a half and two and a half grams of carbs per pound of body weight are recommended per day. Your fiber intake should be between twenty-five and thirty-five grams of fiber per day. Your fiber intake is counted toward your daily total carb intake.

Protein

The last main nutrient on the nutrition label is protein. Protein is used for the growth and repair of cells in the body. There is some debate as to how much is appropriate for a healthy adult to ingest on a daily basis. Many bodybuilders and fitness enthusiasts consider this to be the holy grail of building and repairing their bodies. A healthy adult should aim to consume between three-quarters of a gram and one and a half grams per pound of bodyweight of protein per day. Keep in mind that all of these totals are subject to change depending on your physical needs and demands. It is a good idea to check with a health-care professional or nutritionist before you make any drastic changes.

Vitamins and Minerals

On the bottom of food labels is the vitamins and minerals section, which may be quite long, depending on how nutrient-dense the food is. Many vitamins and minerals are naturally occurring in the food we eat. However, the more processed foods you eat, the less chance you have of consuming these nutrients. It is always best to get your daily requirements from food itself, but choosing a reputable multivitamin and mineral supplement is an acceptable alternative.

Ingredients

The ingredients section is usually listed below the main nutrients section. A lot of the companies may advertise this information elsewhere on the package to show you the value their product offers over others. For instance, the companies offering healthier foods want you to know their product is fat free, is low in carbs, and is approved by the American Heart Association. The non-GMO sign is also growing in popularity, as this means that the food product you are purchasing is not genetically modified. This is a pretty good sign that you are purchasing a healthy product, but be sure to read the label in its entirety. There can still be some hidden ingredients that you should stay away from.

What Else You Should Look For

Processed foods are much more common today than they were years ago. Many people have gotten used to fast foods or microwavable meals because they are quick and convenient. Processed foods are cooked in high amounts of fat and may contain a lot of preservatives and artificial ingredients to increase their shelf life. While they are edible and taste good to many people, they usually lack many of the nutrients the body needs. This may not cause any problems for you right away, but over time your health and physical appearance will begin to take a hit.

It's very easy to ignore a problem you don't know you have. Right now you may be worried that some of your favorite foods are bad for you. This doesn't mean that you have to stop eating them all at once. Quitting cold turkey is a tough thing to do and doesn't work for everyone. The more reasonable approach would be to make smarter decisions and limit the amount of unhealthy food you eat. If you can stop at once, by all means you should do it. Otherwise, begin now by eliminating some of the bad food and replacing it with a more healthy choice. Just because it's healthy does not mean that it will taste bad. Much of the healthy food on the market tastes good. If it did not, food companies would not sell it.

Modified and Hydrogenated Ingredients

Here is an idea of what to look for and avoid when you are out grocery shopping. First, any modified or hydrogenated ingredient means that the product has been processed in some way. If you were to look at the chemical structure of an unsaturated fat and compare it to a bioengineered fat, you would see that the difference between the two is obvious. Hydrogenated oils are heated to very high temperatures and then injected with a catalyst. This increases the density of the oil and changes it from a liquid to a solid at room temperature. It takes the body more time to break down the latter. This robs the body of energy needed for other functions and saps your own energy level for daily activities. Have you ever crashed in the afternoon after eating your lunch and then wondered why? Look to what you ate for the answer. For example, natural peanut butter is better for you than regular peanut butter, because regular peanut butter has hydrogenated oil, which is more difficult to break down and digest. Natural peanut butter tastes just as good, and most people never know the difference. It also does not contain hydrogenated oils.

High-Fructose Corn Syrup

High-fructose corn syrup and other refined sugars should be avoided if possible. There have been studies done on refined sugars that link them to cancer and other diseases in the body. They have also been connected to weight gain. Remember, any excess sugar that is not used up by the body has the potential to be stored as fat. Too much of any carbohydrate can cause this to happen. Refined sugars have been linked to different diseases in the body, the most notable of which is diabetes. There have also been studies that link sugar to inflammation in the body. Inflammation is the beginning stage for many diseases.

People often ask what they can do to look and stay younger. Dr. Mehmet Oz offers useful information about the relationship between sugar and inflammation in the body. His books are great to read and can teach you how to recognize and therefore prevent different disorders. Another notable source to look up is Dr. Nicholas Perricone, who specializes in skin care and looking younger. If you look at the ingredients listed on a can of bread crumbs, you may be surprised to see what goes into the finished product. You should definitely begin to pay attention to this substance if you are not already doing so.

Artificial Sweeteners

Artificial sweeteners are the next category of things to avoid. There is some debate as to how these affect your body. Some people are allergic to these substances, as they can trigger headaches and stomach discomfort. Others say they are not affected at all. Artificial sweeteners and preservatives have become so common that it's sometimes challenging to find a packaged food without them. Pay close attention to the ingredients section. Sweeteners such as sucralose, NutraSweet, acesulfame potassium, and aspartame are artificial. Try to replace these with stevia. Stevia, also known as Rebiana, is a natural sweetener that comes from a plant.

Preservatives

Preservatives have been added to and used in food for a long time. There are natural and chemical food preservatives. Natural preservatives, such as sugar, salt, vinegar, and alcohol, are commonly used for pickling, juices, and jams. Fresh meats and fish are also preserved with salt. Canned goods like soup can be dehydrated, and coffee can be freeze-dried. Buying foods in an airtight sealed package is another natural way to add some longevity to your grocery stockpile.

Chemical preservatives, including benzoates, sulfites, nitrates, and sorbates, are another way food is kept fresh. These chemicals do keep food fresh for longer periods of time, but some have been proven to be harmful. The long-term use of sulfur dioxide and nitrates is a suspected cause of cancer. Allergies and skin rashes have also been linked to certain preservatives. Until the food companies can find a better way or are banned from using these substances, you must be careful not to ingest too many chemical preservatives. To protect yourself and your family, you should limit the amount of these substances as much as possible. Other preservatives to look out for are propionic acid, sorbic acid, benzoic acid, caramel, butylated hydroxyanisol (BHA), and butylates.

Fat-Free Products

Another thing you should consider on your next grocery trip has to do with fat-free products. For instance, the dairy section has several foods that are fat free. These products are naturally fat free and are not chemically altered. But foods that naturally contain fat and carry a fat-free label may have been altered in some way. Fat free does not necessarily mean that it is good for you. Consider this for a moment: if a product like mayo normally has ten grams of fat but the fat has been removed, what has it been replaced with? Most likely it is either a lot sugar or a filler of some sort to keep the original appearance and consistency.

The filler is most likely an artificial ingredient. Fat can be digested by the body, but can the artificial ingredients and fillers be broken down? That is debatable. If regular mayo is used in moderation, it should not be a problem for you. If you eat it like a cup of yogurt, you might want to rethink your strategy. Consuming food products with naturally-occurring ingredients is the best and safest way to go.

Now that you know how to interpret nutrition labels, shopping should make much more sense. It may take a little while to get adjusted and apply what you are learning, but pretty soon you will be an expert and be able to explain these concepts to your friends and family. When you understand why you are doing something a certain way, you will have a better chance of sticking with it.

How to Grocery Shop

One should eat to live, not live to eat.

— BENJAMIN FRANKLIN

It Begins with Produce

The entrance to most grocery stores will be near the produce section. Fresh fruits and vegetables are extremely important and necessary for proper health. They contain many vitamins, minerals, antioxidants, carbs, fiber, and other nutrients the body needs. The suggested amount of vegetables a healthy adult should consume on a daily basis is two and a half to three cups per day. The suggested amount of fruit is about two cups per day, depending on how physically active you are. Those who have a physically demanding job, play sports, and exercise on a daily basis can consume more.

There are many vegetables to choose from. For your convenience, here is a list of common choices:

- artichokes
- asparagus
- acorn squash
- bean sprouts
- beets
- brussels sprouts
- butternut squash
- broccoli
- cabbage
- cauliflower
- celery
- cucumbers
- carrots
- collard greens
- eggplant
- green beans
- lettuce (different kinds)
- mushrooms
- mustard greens

- onions
- okra
- peas
- peppers
- spinach
- sweet potatoes
- tomatoes
- turnips
- turnip greens
- white potatoes
- wax beans
- zucchini

There are even more to choose from. Don't be afraid to try something new. Your taste buds can change over time, and what you did not like before may satisfy you now.

There are many different ways to prepare your vegetables. Enjoying them raw is usually the most nutritious way to eat them. However, some taste much better after they have been cooked. It is a personal preference. The best way to prepare your vegetables and get the most out of them is to steam them. Using the grill or the oven are the other preferred methods of cooking. You should try to avoid boiling your veggies, as you will end up cooking out a lot of the nutrients. Unless you are using the water they are cooked in for a broth, you should avoid boiling them. The microwave is also a common way to cook vegetables that should be avoided. Using the microwave may denature the vegetable, making it not as nutritious.

Buying your vegetables fresh is the best way to ensure you are getting a quality product. If you can afford to go organic, you should do so. It only costs a few dollars more. Try to avoid buying the frozen, canned, or processed vegetables. These may not be as nutrient-dense as the fresh produce that is available. Remember, the preferred methods of cooking vegetables are steaming them, baking them in the oven, or eating them raw.

The recommendations for fruit are similar to those for vegetables. Most fruit is eaten raw, but if you do cook fruit, you should use the oven or stove top. Limit yourself from using the microwave if possible because of the denaturing effect it may have. Fresh fruit is better than the canned or frozen kind. If you do need to buy the canned variety, check the food label to avoid buying a product with extra sugar added. The same applies to juices. Natural and organic varieties are available and are definitely the better choice.

There are a variety of fruits to choose from. For your convenience, here is a list of common choices:

- apples
- apricots
- avocados
- bananas
- blueberries
- cherries
- cantaloupe
- grapefruit
- grapes
- honeydew melons
- kiwis
- lemons
- limes
- mangoes
- nectarines
- oranges
- peaches
- pears

- plums
- papayas
- pineapples
- prunes
- raisins
- strawberries
- raspberries
- tangerines

The Organic Section

As previously mentioned, organic fruits and vegetables are supposed to be the healthier way to go for produce. This is because fertilizers and other possibly harmful chemicals are not used on them. Pesticides and other chemicals are also not used, keeping the fruits and vegetables more clean and natural. This section in the store is mixed in with the produce department. Most likely, an additional section featuring all types of organic products is located next to or near the produce department. Although a bit more demanding on your pocketbook, organic foods come with peace of mind, as you can be assured that you are getting the most natural products available. There are people who will claim that they only shop organic. Whatever your decision, you at least have the choice.

To save money on organic groceries, try visiting a local farmers market. Sometimes this is only possible in the summertime or when certain produce is in season. Pay attention to local growers who set up stands on the side of the road to sell their crops. If you are driving on the road and see a sign for locally grown produce, you should stop and check it out. You may get lucky and find a few more good deals you were not expecting.

Some farmers even have special deals allowing you to pay one lump sum and receive fresh produce for the whole summer.

The Delicious Deli

The deli section is very popular for many reasons. The food available there can provide a quick meal, and it tastes good and is affordable, especially if there is a sale going on (and there is almost always a sale). There are a few things you should consider when picking out your favorite selections. Always check the nutrition label on the product you are purchasing. Fat, sodium, cholesterol, and preservatives are your main concern. Some things are unavoidable, which is why you should limit your deli intake.

There are certain brands that make a much cleaner product. Dietz and Watson is a well-known brand that aims to reduce fat, cholesterol, sodium, and preservatives while providing a good source of protein. This is a great combination for the health-conscious shopper. Even though this brand is healthier than other deli selections, regular meat is still the best way to go. If you have a local Giant Eagle, the Market District brand is also a much healthier way to go.

The deli section may also include some prepared foods and complete meals. The better your understanding of nutrition and the more familiar you are with nutrition labels, the more likely you will be to make an educated decision about what you should choose. For instance, you may choose the three-bean salad over the coleslaw, because the beans have less fat. If you have not eaten much fat that day but are close to your daily intake of sodium, you would choose the coleslaw. Both are a good choice; your selection should depend on what else you ate that day.

Super Seafood

Seafood is a great choice to make when you are looking to eat healthier. You want to make sure that you only consume fish about three times per week. Although fish is usually high in protein and low in fat, there is concern that too much can be bad for you. It does contain a certain amount of heavy metals and pollutants that you need to stay away from. A list of common types of fish may include:

- cod
- crab
- flounder
- haddock
- halibut
- lobster
- mahimahi
- salmon
- sardines
- scallops
- shrimp
- swordfish
- trout
- tilapia
- tuna

Salmon contains more fat than regular fish but is very high in omega-3 fatty acids, which are a super nutrient for the body. If you are able to, purchase the wild caught Alaskan salmon. There are many health benefits to eating seafood, as it can lower your cholesterol levels and improve your heart function, and it is also good for your joints. There are several ways to prepare and enjoy seafood. To be safe, you should purchase seafood from a reputable market or restaurant.

The Meat Section

Meat is a great source of protein, vitamins, and minerals. The meat section offers a wide variety of choices for healthy eating. You do want to be careful which grade of meat you select. Fat content can range anywhere from as low as about 2 percent up to 30 percent and higher. Generally speaking, the leaner the meat is, the better it is for you. Red meat usually has a higher fat content compared to most poultry. Chicken breast is an example of a meat that is high in protein and very low in fat. To avoid the slightly higher price tag on lean meats, you should wait to purchase it until it is on sale. You can then buy it in bulk and freeze it to save money. Some common meat choices are:

- beef
- bison
- chicken
- lamb
- liver
- turkey
- veal
- venison

Check the date on the package to make sure you can use or freeze the meat in the time period allotted. Some meats keep longer than others, and you don't want to waste your money on something you will not be able to eat.

The Dairy Section

The dairy section is usually located somewhere near the back of the store. When shopping for dairy products, you need to be mindful of what you're looking for in a healthy food. Some of the advice in the previous pages may not hold true for dairy products. Milk, for example, is a good source of protein but can be high in sugar and fat. Usually you would want to avoid high sugar and fat, but this is not true of milk. This does not mean you can drink all the milk you want and not have to pay the consequences. Depending on what your meal plan looks like, one of the several choices of milk that are available will be acceptable, from skim to whole milk. Some may say that skim is the way to go because it's fat free. Others may tell you that the digestive enzymes found in whole milk are beneficial, as they help you absorb more of the healthy nutrients. If you choose whole milk, keep track of how much you consume, so it does not become a problem.

Aside from regular milk products, the dairy section now offers several alternatives, such as almond milk, rice milk, Lactaid, and other choices. Many people have allergies to dairy products but still want to drink milk, and there are a number of available alternatives. They are healthy alternatives that also give you a little bit of variety.

Yogurt is another example of a food that is good for you but also may contain some unwanted sugar. Yogurt is not only a good source of protein, it also contains active cultures that aid in your digestion. Do not skip on yogurt just because of the sugar content. Keep in mind that some of these products may use artificial sweeteners to keep the sugar content to a minimum. It's up to you if you want to eat it or not. Your best bet would be to choose the plain-flavored yogurt, because it does not have a bunch of added sugar. Not every food choice will be clear-cut. Take a moment before you decide and then choose what you feel is your best option.

Cheese is the next food that, depending on how it is used, can be good or bad. Cottage cheese may be your best choice. It is a good source of protein and calcium. You can decide between the high- and low-fat varieties. They also make low-sodium varieties that may be of interest to those who need to watch their sodium intake.

One of the best foods in the dairy section is the almighty egg. The egg has been called nature's perfect food. It is high in protein, vitamins, and minerals. It was once thought that the amount of cholesterol in an egg was bad for you, but new studies have proven that this is not the case. The cholesterol in eggs does not have the same impact on the body as the cholesterol from other sources does. This doesn't mean you should eat all the yolks you can, but don't feel bad if you do eat a few of the yolks. Whether you like them hard-boiled or sunny-side up, eggs should be a part of your daily meal plan. Some common dairy items are:

- milk
- yogurt
- eggs
- cheese
- cream
- butter

Although butter is mostly fat, it is an ingredient in just about every recipe. Selecting real butter over many of the spreads may be a better choice. You should use butter in moderation to avoid consuming too much fat.

Frozen Foods

The frozen foods section has just about any food you can think of. Fresh is best, but frozen will work for the busy individual. You can make a lot of good purchases here; you just need to read the labels and know what you are looking for. Frozen foods tend to contain a lot of sodium and fat. The high sodium content is part of the preserving process that helps make these foods last longer. To most people, it also makes the food taste better. Salt has a way of bringing out the flavor that may otherwise be a bit bland. This is good for the companies making money selling their products but is not as good for someone who is maintaining a more healthy meal plan.

Many of the companies have designed options that are lower in fat, sodium, and cholesterol. The protein content is usually high, but the quality may be questionable due to the source of the protein. After reading and comparing a few different nutrition labels, you should start to get a pretty good idea of what you should choose. New products are hitting the shelves all the time, making it difficult to say which would be the best choice. You really have to look and compare on this one.

Lean Cuisine is a good example of a frozen entrée that may suit the needs of healthy individuals. Healthy Request is another good brand you can find in the frozen food section. Taste should not be much of a concern, as it is unlikely that the company would put out a bland product. The grocery store you shop at may even have its own brand of healthy foods. Apply what you are learning and keep your eye out for the most sensible choice.

The In-Between Aisles

At this point the rest of your shopping will take place in the center of the store. The aisles in the middle contain many of the food groups already discussed; however, in these aisles the food choices are packaged in boxes or cans. This is where you have to be very careful about what you choose to eat. There is much more temptation to pick up desserts, potato chips, and other snacks that contain not-so-good-for-you ingredients.

When choosing any kind of grain or carbohydrate, make sure to avoid things like high-fructose corn syrup and bleached products. Preservatives and artificial sweeteners are also more likely to be included in the foods in these aisles. Pasta, bread, cereal, crackers, chips, cookies, and other boxed and miscellaneous canned items are all located in the middle aisles of the store. There are still many good choices to make when walking these aisles; you just need to read the labels carefully.

The Fillers Category

This category includes many of the things shoppers commonly include in their grocery carts. Since you have taken the initiative to make better decisions about your health, you will recognize what is good for you and what is not. Making healthier and more educated decisions should be a part of your daily routine. This new daily routine is going to payoff exponentially in the long run.

The fillers category includes items such as cookies, chips, ice cream, candy, pastries, and any other highly processed products. Items that are mass-produced to meet the demands of the market are generally filled with a bunch of preservatives and refined sugars. If you eat these products only on special occasions, chances are you will not be affected. However, many people eat these items as part of their daily diet. Then they wonder why they are out of shape and have no energy. Common sense tells you that this cannot be good for you.

If you are one of those individuals who have to have their sugar and salt fix, you may have to work a little harder to fix the impediment. Do not worry; you can overcome it. Foods like cookies and ice cream can be addicting because of the high sugar content. Breaking this habit is possible if you are committed to improving your health and being more financially secure. Your eating habits are psychological and are a representation of how you think of your body. Different techniques and suggestions will be discussed later to help you overcome these obstacles.

The Perimeter Is Best

You may have noticed that most of the healthier food choices are found around the perimeter of the store. It's almost as if the stores were designed to give shoppers the benefit of making healthy selections, beginning with the produce section and wrapping all the way around to the cash registers. It's a very logical and smooth design that makes things easier for the inexperienced healthy shopper. No matter where you shop, the layout should be similar. In case of an exception, you should still be prepared and able to understand how to shop for the right groceries. The information laid out in this book provides you with the resources to make the appropriate choices for good health.

To be the most efficient shopper you can be, stick to the perimeter first, then weave in and out of the aisles. The idea is to fill up your cart with the good stuff, then pick up the remainder of whatever else you may want or need. Imagine that your grocery cart is divided into sections: carbohydrates, protein, healthy fats, fiber, produce, personal items, and fillers. Fulfilling these main nutritional requirements will be a huge part of your success. Anything extra in your cart may fall into the fillers category, meaning you just don't need it.

Take the time to review this information frequently so you are familiar with the content and know what to look for when you are grocery shopping. After a while, you will begin to remember which food is acceptable and which food you should stay away from. You may even begin to memorize some food labels and nutrition facts. This is a good sign that you are retaining much of the information presented here, which will help you make better decisions when you eat out at a restaurant. Continue to explore new products and look for any changes companies may make on their nutrition labels. It doesn't happen too often, but sometimes the information does change. With this mind-set, a successful trip to the grocery store is only a few moments away.

Dining Out

Your life is busy, and you may not always be able to prepare every single meal ahead of time. When the weekend is here and you want to just sit around and relax after a long work week, cooking dinner may be the last thing on your mind. Whatever your excuse or reason may be, it is completely unacceptable… just kidding. Dining out is something everyone does.

Your general knowledge about nutrition will help you make healthier choices. Most restaurants are familiar with and cater to fit-conscious patrons. From salads to low-calorie entrées, there is something on the menu for everyone. If the restaurant you are eating at does not offer low-calorie options, use your best judgment as to what you think is healthy. Here are twelve things to consider when eating out:

1. Thin crust is healthier than regular crust.
2. Grilled food is better than fried food.
3. Shed half the bun and enjoy an open-faced sandwich.
4. Choose a baked potato over fries.
5. Sweet potatoes or yams are better than regular baked potatoes.

6. Salad and steamed vegetables are the most nutritious options.
7. Ask for low-calorie dressing or just use vinegar and a small amount of oil.
8. Sweetened drinks usually contain high amounts of sugar.
9. Water is calorie free (just add lemon).
10. Dessert is not necessary.
11. Ask that no salt be added to your food if possible.
12. If you are craving flavor, try spicy instead of salty.

This should give you a good idea of how to eat when you are away from home and not in control of cooking the meal. Do not be afraid to tell the waiter how you want your food prepared. In fact, your server may even suggest some healthy specials that are available. This is becoming more and more common, depending on where you dine out.

With the invention of smartphones, people have become quite savvy at looking things up on a dime. With several different applications available to help you make healthier choices, it has become easier to dine out. There are specific applications that will give you the breakdown of the nutritional information at the restaurant of your choice. In fact, if you visit the company's website, you may be able to view the nutritional information right there.

Eat This or That

Let's say you have been at work all day and have done everything right in the nutrition department. On your way home, you decide to stop at McDonald's for dinner. Keeping in mind you want to eat healthier, you decide to order a chicken salad with

Italian dressing on the side. This may not be as healthy as you think. A few things to consider are the dressing and the chicken. Depending on what kind of chicken and dressing they are using, the meal may be high in fat and sodium.

Restaurants obtain the ingredients for their food from different sources. Similar to deli meats, the chicken may be highly processed and not easily broken down by your body, unlike regular store-bought chicken. After eating, if you feel like your food is sitting in your stomach for an extra long time, chances are it was a highly processed meal. You should know what a normal piece of grilled chicken looks like. If the chicken on your salad does not look like regular chicken, but instead looks like something that was squeezed out of a tube, you should probably consider the source. It's still going to be edible and does contain protein, but it's not as nutritious as the kind bought from the store or farm.

When it comes to dressings, some contain high amounts of fat and sodium. The dressings they give you from restaurants may contain as much as twenty-two grams of fat per serving. You also need to pay attention to the amount of servings per packet. What you think is only one serving may really be two. Now twenty-two grams of fat quickly becomes forty-four grams of fat; so much for the healthy meal. Always ask for the healthiest dressing they have. If the person serving you does not have the answer, ask to compare the dressings or make your best educated guess.

In this situation it should be very clear that going home to cook your chicken on the grill and choosing your own healthy dressing is the better way to go. Do the best that you can in whatever circumstance you're in. If you have to stop at a fast-food place, at least you'll be aware of the challenges you are going to face. Ordering chicken salad from a fast-food establishment is still much better than ordering two or three hamburgers with fries.

What About Taste?

A very common concern many people have about healthy eating is about the taste of food. People believe that if they eat healthy, it's not going to taste good. With that in mind, they decide that eating healthy is going to be boring and tortuous. This is a pretty legitimate concern but could not be further from the truth. You should be enjoying the process of getting in shape, not dreading it.

It is a fact that some people eat bland food when they are trying to lose weight. It is a very boring plan for losing weight when a few boiled chicken breasts, salad with no dressing, and water are the only things on the menu. However, this is not a requirement and is not recommended. In order for you to successfully enjoy a healthy lifestyle, eating tasty food is a necessity. If you were expected to eat only bland food, you would probably not be able keep up with your goals for very long. Even the bodybuilders and fitness models understand this. You need to include some sort of variety.

When they are cutting weight, most professionals do eat smaller portions and are very careful not to add anything that would inhibit their progress. Through trial and error, many clever and flavorful recipes have been created to help support fitness enthusiasts' goal of fat loss and lean muscle development. Sitting down to a good meal is something that everyone appreciates. Your success will be much greater when you develop a sense of balance in your nutrition plan.

It does help to know your way around the kitchen. You do not have to be a gourmet chef, but a little cookbook knowledge can go a long way. If you cook on a regular basis, this should be easy for you. If you are new to cooking, this is nothing to be concerned about. As long as you can read and follow directions, you will be able to whip up a healthy treat in no time. If you are interested in learning how to cook, you could always take a cooking class. And depending on your financial situation, perhaps hiring an in-home cook or chef is an option.

Supplements

In order to meet the higher demands you will be putting on your body, you may need to take supplements to ensure you are getting all the essential vitamins and nutrients. If you eat well-balanced meals, you should be able to get most of these nutrients. However, for most people, finding the time to cook and prepare the right foods while staying on track can be very challenging. It may be especially time-consuming if you are also juggling family, work, and exhaustion. This is in no way, shape, or form an excuse for you to skip out on good nutrition, but it is a real concern. So how do you fix it?

Ever since the fitness lifestyle first began to get recognition, people have been looking for quick and healthy solutions to feed their bodies between meals and during workouts. With time and nutrition being the main concern, people began embracing the idea of supplements. Taking vitamin and mineral supplements became popular to help fill the void for people who did not eat enough of the right foods. This would also be a solution to another problem. With the invention of mass-produced and processed foods, the nutrition content was starting to take a hit. This meant that many of the essential nutrients that people used to get from certain foods were now lacking, and the food was not as nutritious. Supplements were created to address this issue.

The dietary needs of an individual who plays sports and exercises are greater than those of a sedentary person, and supplements help active people maintain a solid nutrition plan. For example, if you are very physically active, protein shakes and meal replacement powders (MRPs) are a great way to ingest the calories and nutrients that you need quickly. They are easily transported and can be taken with you wherever you go, making them an essential item to keep in the pantry.

Depending on what your physical and nutritional goals are, there are several kinds of supplements you can take. Keep in mind that you don't have to take any supplements if you don't want to. In fact, some people are against supplementing and believe they can get everything they need from the food they eat. This may have been the case several years ago, but with today's food supplies being mass-produced and processed, the nutritional value may not be what it once was. Processed foods are definitely not that high in nutritional value. Certain crops are being grown and harvested at such a fast pace that the soil that supports these crops does not have the time to recover properly to be as nutrient-dense as possible.

Food is still believed by many to be the best way to get your nutrients. Supplements are supposed to be just that—a supplement. They are not supposed to completely replace food, but instead are designed to help give you a boost in certain areas in which you are lacking good nutrition. The topic of supplements can be talked about in much greater detail. This section was included to give you a brief introduction into the world of supplementation. Supplements will be discussed more in the training section of this book.

Antioxidants

Antioxidants are the protectors of the body. They help to fight off free radicals and other potentially harmful substances in the body. To give you a better example of what a free radical is and how much it affects your body, consider the following. When you take a bite of an apple and let it sit on the counter for a few minutes, what happens? The apple will start to turn brown and begin to rot. Oxygen is considered a free radical and actually begins to break down the apple. Antioxidants like vitamins A, C, and E and ECGC (green tea extract) help to prevent this process. It obviously does not happen as fast in your body, but at least you have a better understanding of what free radicals do and how to protect against them.

pH Balance

Your body is constantly working to keep you healthy and productive. In fact, your body is constantly maintaining your pH balance. The pH scale ranges from being acidic to being alkaline. To maintain your body's homeostasis (balance), your pH level should be around 7.3 or 7.4. If your body falls out of this range, serious injury and even death can occur.

Everything you eat has a pH balance. It is very difficult to fall out of the optimal range, but different stomach and gastrointestinal issues can arise from an unbalanced diet. Many of the processed foods people eat are more on the acidic side. Have you ever eaten a large meal and suffered from heartburn afterward? Most people can relate to this example. It may have been something that you ate. Maybe the food was more acidic than you thought.

It is much better to be on the alkaline side of things than the acidic side. Studies have shown that individuals who eat alkaline diets are less likely to develop and suffer from disease. There have even been instances in which people claimed to have healed themselves from cancer by eating such a diet, though they made some other changes in their life, as well. The food you consume has a lot to do with your overall health. This is definitely something to take seriously. Fruits and vegetables are considered to be more alkaline. Processed foods, grains, and meat are considered to be more acidic. Here is a list of some alkaline foods you should make sure to fit into your nutrition plan:

- avocados
- alfalfa
- apples
- bananas
- blueberries
- cranberries
- cucumbers
- lemons
- limes
- okra
- raspberries
- strawberries
- spinach
- wheatgrass
- watermelon

You probably recognize a pattern here. A lot of the fruits and vegetables in our diets are more on the alkaline side of the scale. That is why it is so important to include vegetables and greens in all of your meals. Carbs, proteins, and fats are not balanced without the company of greens and vegetables.

Timing Your Meals

Food is fuel and needs to be looked at as such. When someone tries to get into the right frame of mind for starting a diet, a few things may happen. The first three letters in diet are d-i-e, which spells die. People can mentally kill their chances of success by trying to stay strict with a diet. When you go on a diet, you are suddenly making a drastic change that will not go unnoticed by your body, which will respond with cravings. Some people can do this and follow through without any problems, but many more people have issues staying on track with the plan. Rather than starting a hard-core diet, it may be more beneficial for you to slowly adopt a healthier and more mentally sound way of choosing your nutrition. Fuel up your body, don't just eat. Your body depends on food for energy to function on a daily basis. If you do not supply your body with the fuel it needs when it needs it, you may suffer from one or more of these five consequences:

1. Lack of energy
2. Unsatisfied appetite and thirst
3. Weight gain
4. Muscle atrophy or muscle breakdown
5. Slower metabolism

You should not eat a lot of food late in the evening before you go to bed, as it can be rather uncomfortable lying down with a belly full of food. It also can be harder to fall into a deep sleep and get sufficient rest. If you were not aware of this before, now you know. Some people also get into the habit of skipping breakfast in the morning, claiming they don't have time or are simply not hungry. Let's say you did not eat anything after 8:00 p.m. and you woke up the next morning at 6:00 a.m. and skipped breakfast. If you are like many people, you may drink coffee and think of it as your first meal. There are not any calories in coffee unless you add in milk, cream, or sugar. If you do not eat your first solid meal until 11:00 a.m., you have just gone fifteen hours without feeding your body! When you wait this long between meals, your body still has to produce energy for you to function. Even when you are fast asleep in your bed, your body still needs energy for basic functions, such as breathing and maintaining your heartbeat.

In order for your body to produce and maintain itself with such a lack of nutrients, it has to break down stored energy. After your body uses any extra glucose and fat deposits in the blood, it looks for another source of fuel. At this point your body believes you are trying to starve it and it must do something to protect you. With no carbohydrates or sugars available for energy, your body will digest and use protein instead. This protein comes from your hard-earned and desirable muscle. Your body breaks down muscle into protein, which can then be converted into the energy you need for normal bodily functions. This puts you into a catabolic state, which means your muscles are breaking down and not being supported. In the long run, this will hurt your ability to shed unwanted weight and keep fit. Remember, the more lean muscle mass you have, the more able you are to burn fat and stay in shape.

If you are one of those people who only eat one or two meals a day, you too are putting your metabolism at risk. Your body will believe it should operate in more of a famine-type state. This means that when you eat, instead of burning up calories for regular consumption, your body will actually work to store them. This can cause weight gain. Your body is trying to ready itself to last a longer period of time, since the proper nutrients and fuel are not coming in on a regular basis. This is a good thing if you get stranded on a desert island but is bad if you are trying keep muscle and stay fit. Since you are not fueling your body appropriately when you skip meals, you can also put your body into a catabolic state.

In theory you are wasting muscle. When your body has to digest muscle for energy, its natural ability to burn and metabolize calories decreases. This can cause you to gain unnecessary fat. If you already have a high level of muscle mass to begin with, your body can last longer without putting on the extra weight, but you will still lose your muscle mass. The more muscle you have, the more efficient you are at burning off fat, so it does not accumulate in your body. If you skip meals or fail to time your meals appropriately, you may gain weight and have a more difficult time reaching your goals.

Much of this depends on whether you have a slow or fast metabolism. This is where your age can make a difference. The older people are, the more likely their metabolism will slow down. However, the more in shape they are, the better chance they stand at keeping their metabolism high and staying fit. The earlier you start to do this, the better your long-term results will be.

Think about investing money into a Roth or a retirement account. The experts will tell you that the earlier you start, the more money you will have in the end. This is because your account is going to earn interest and compound interest over the years. If you start to invest at age twenty-five and do not retire until age sixty, you have quite a long time to add up your investments and let the interest build, yielding you a much more rewarding return.

On the other hand, if you did not start investing until you were fifty years old and retired at age sixty, there is no way you would be able to invest the same amount of money as you would if you had started when you were younger. You will still have money in the bank that is earning interest that you can retire on, though not as much. The same principle applies for investing in your health and fitness. The earlier you start to invest in yourself and take pride in your health and appearance, the happier and more fulfilled you will be. Here are a few reasons why:

- You will have more energy and endurance.
- You will age more gracefully.
- You will feel better about yourself.
- You will have more confidence.
- You will be presented with more opportunities.
- You will be more of a leader than a follower.

The importance of fitness is universally recognized. You could have every material thing in the world one could ask for but you would not be able to fully enjoy it unless you were healthy. Your health is a gift; please do not take it for granted.

Meal Plan 101

This section will give you an idea of what a healthy meal plan should look like for someone who is trying to develop lean muscle mass and trim excess fat. Every person's plan is going to look a little bit different at first. Instead of going to extremes and changing your foods all at once, it might be better to start out with a couple-day grace period. On the other hand, you may find it easier to just jump right in. Only you know your personality type. If you are honest with yourself, you will see much greater results. Cheating and procrastinating will not get you anywhere. If you want to reach your goal of a better you, start as soon as possible and do not put it off until tomorrow.

Let's say that you wake up at 5:45 a.m. The first thing you are going to want to do is eat breakfast. Breakfast is the most important meal of the day. You are literally breaking the fast after a decent night's rest. Always think about your meals as fuel for the body. The best fuel you can use is a mixture of protein, carbs, and healthy fats. Just eating carbs or just eating protein should be avoided if possible. You want to make sure to group your nutrients together, instead of eating them separately. This will ensure that the foods are digested well and will help to keep your blood sugar at a more consistent level; otherwise, it may spike and cause unwanted fat storage. You always want to be thinking about maintaining a proper balance. If you are in a hurry in the morning, a good quick breakfast to try is a protein shake. In a blender, you can mix one cup of skim milk or water, one scoop of whey (or your choice) protein powder, one tablespoon of natural peanut butter, one small banana, and one cup of ice. This is a fast, easy, and healthy breakfast that tastes great and is portable too!

You should aim to fuel your body every three hours or so to keep nutrients at a healthy level and to ensure you maintain a higher metabolism. Yes, you did read that correctly! You will actually be eating more to lose weight. You do not have to starve yourself like most diets would have you believe. Since 8:45 a.m. is a bit too early for a lunch break, snacking is going to be a good option. An example of a quick snack is one cup of Greek yogurt and a handful of almonds or blueberries. This will give your body the protein, carbs, and healthy fat that you need to keep things running smoothly.

At 11:45 a.m. it is time for lunch. Instead of going out to eat and spending more money than you probably want to, you should pack your lunch and bring it with you. You can pick up a thermal cooler to keep your food cold from just about any Walmart or household goods store. A great lunch to pack would be an albacore tuna wrap with fresh vegetables and low-fat dressing. Drinking water with a packet of naturally sweetened Crystal Light should satisfy your craving for anything sweet. If you are still hungry, you can eat a small bag of baby carrots or whole grain wheat crackers or a small cup of yogurt or mixed fruit.

At 2:45 p.m. you can have another snack. Just add water or skim milk to a shaker bottle filled with one or two scoops of protein powder. You can also eat a handful of almonds to really curb your hunger if you need to.

Dinnertime is right around 5:45 p.m. This is the meal where you can eat well and enjoy it. A good source of protein, like salmon, chicken breast, lean beef, or turkey, is important. Couple that with some steamed or raw vegetables and a healthy carb to complete the meal. Sweet potatoes, yams, or brown rice are some good healthy carbohydrates. Since you will most likely be at home for this meal, you have the flexibility to eat what you want. You do not have to worry about packing anything at this point, unless you have a job where you work late or overnight. In that case, meal preparation is going to be your secret weapon in your quest for a better body.

At 8:45 p.m. it is time for the last meal of the day. Try to give yourself about an hour or so before you lay down after eating. For this snack, you will want to keep your protein high and carbs low and include a small amount of healthy fat. If you choose to go with a protein shake, you should use casein instead of whey. Casein protein is more slowly digested and stays in the blood stream longer, which is good for overnight fasting. Another good choice would be low-fat cottage cheese with some blueberries. Low-fat cottage cheese is high in protein and low in carbs, and the protein it contains is also a slower digesting protein, which makes it good to have in the evening. Since you will be going to bed shortly after this last meal, make sure to keep it as light as possible.

A Few Reminders

Here are a couple of things to remember when picking out your foods. When you select a protein, you want to make sure it is a whole food protein with the least amount of fat. Lean beef, bison, chicken, and turkey are great choices. One exception you can make is salmon, as it is rich in omega-3 fatty acids. These are the good kind of fats that your body needs and that are necessary for many bodily and hormonal functions. If you are going to use a supplement such as whey protein, pick out a product that lists the typical amino acid profile. This is a good indication that it is a quality product and that your body is going to get the nutrients it needs.

When selecting your carbs, you need to be smart and pick out the healthier choice. Think of it this way: if you pour water on a carbohydrate source and it swells, it is most likely going to swell in your body. Swelling causes inflammation, and inflammation is a leading cause for disease and other illnesses. This is not to say that bad carbs are going to make you sick and cause disease, but there is a lot of published literature relating sugar to illnesses and ailments in the body. The most notable of them is diabetes insipidus. It would be wise to do some further research on this subject. White bread, pasta, and white rice will swell when you add water to them, whereas carrots, almonds, yams, and bananas will not, or at least not to the same degree. Now think about what they are going to do inside your body and you should get the picture. If it doesn't swell on the outside, it probably won't swell on the inside.

When you think of balance and keeping your nutrients in check, think of vegetables, as they offer the body a wide variety of benefits. Vegetables are live foods filled with enzymes and many other beneficial and protective substances that help to prevent and fight disease. They are full of vitamins, minerals, and antioxidants and are a good source of fiber. Most vegetables are also more alkaline and are good for cleansing the body and keeping things regular and consistent.

Fats are another very important nutrient that your body needs and cannot function without. Fats are needed for many bodily and hormonal functions. They also help lubricate your joints and promote healthy skin and a healthy cardiovascular system. The omega fats found in nuts, fish, and vegetables should be a mainstay in your diet.

These points are being repeated several times in this book to help you remember them. You want to look at food as the fuel and energy needed for the body to perform at its peak physical condition. Remember the sports car analogy? The rarest, fastest, and longest-lasting car is going to require the most premium fuel, because it burns the cleanest and is not loaded up with fillers and junk the engine doesn't need. That would only cause the engine to stall and run poorly. In this case, longevity and quality are equal to intelligence and purity. Know it, practice it, live it, and become it. You will see and feel the difference in everything you do.

Sample Meal Plan

5:45 a.m.	1 cup skim milk or water, 1 scoop whey protein, 1 tbs of natural peanut butter, 1 small banana, and 1 cup of ice blended together
8:45 a.m.	1 cup of Greek yogurt, 1 handful of almonds or blue berries
11:45 a.m.	1 can albacore tuna, 1 low-carb or spinach wrap, fresh spinach and red pepper slices, 2 tbs low-fat mayo (or substitute Greek yogurt) and 1 small bag of carrots or 1 cup of natural applesauce
2:45 p.m.	1 cup skim milk or water, 1 scoop whey protein mixed together, and a handful of almonds or blueberries
5:45 p.m.	1 chicken breast or piece of salmon, 1 cooked yam, and 2 cups of steamed vegetables
8:45 p.m.	1 cup low-fat cottage cheese with a handful of berries

*Note: As for beverages, water is the most important liquid you should be consuming. Your body is made up of mostly water; on average 60-72 percent. Most alternative beverages on the market contain a lot of sugar and other unnecessary fillers and additives. If you are really craving some flavor and need to have something different, try the naturally flavored Crystal Light packets they sell at the grocery store. Crystal Light now has a product that uses stevia, instead of the artificial sweeteners many other beverages use. It is very low calorie and tastes pretty good.

Take a Look at Paleo

The paleo nutrition plan is gaining a wide acceptance as of late. The idea behind paleo is that you are only supposed to eat foods that are natural and from the earth. Another name for it is the *caveman diet*. The paleo plan excludes processed foods, sugars, almost all if not all dairy, and anything that is genetically modified to make a whole food unnatural. Beans, soy, and peanuts may also be on the do-not-eat list because of the chemical responses they produce in your body.

Have you ever noticed that certain foods you eat can make you very bloated and flatulent? It is either because you have an allergy, you lack the proper enzymes to digest and break the food down properly, or it contains something artificial and should not have been ingested in the first place. For example, corn, oats, wheat, and other bread products are not considered paleo under some nutrition plans. The reason is that most forms of this agriculture have been genetically modified or processed in some way. Experts are even going as far to say that we may never get back to nature's intended makeup of these products. That is a pretty harsh statement and very sad to think about, but with all of the tampering of our food supply and all of the chemical additives included to make food supposedly last longer, it's no wonder why. For years, the FDA and developers have said that the food is safe and that they would not be allowed to make it any other way. And for years, there have been documented cases and studies that supposedly prove many of these additives and preservatives are harmful in some way.

Now, this should not be taken as gospel. Any of the ideas in this book can be challenged. It would be wise to do some deeper research into this subject and see what you can come up with. Some of the information in this section plays devil's advocate to some of the information laid out for you earlier, but you will learn through trial and error what does and does not work for you. There are some foods you will be able to eat without incident. There may be some foods that will not agree with your body and should be avoided. Make sure to keep a good journal of your discoveries and progress along the way. For more relevant information regarding this and other topics, please visit www.fitenomics.com and look over the articles and nutrition sections. There are some great paleo recipes worth looking into that help lay the foundation for this idea.

One More Thing

There are many different ways to eat healthily. The ideas presented in this book are for your general health and well-being. Each individual person is going to have different micronutrient and macronutrient requirements. For example, if you decide you want to look like a bodybuilder, you will not get there by making healthy food choices alone; that is not going to be enough. You will need to be very specific about what and when you eat to keep your hormones at the optimal levels to reach your full potential.

A great reference to read regarding this subject is *Macrobolic Nutrition* by Gerard Dente and Kevin J. Hopkins. After years of competing and researching the subject of nutrition, they have come up with a formula of 45 percent carbs, 35 percent protein, and 20 percent fat to keep your body in the most anabolic state. They suggest eating every two and a half to three hours to keep levels at their peak. It is important to stay as close as possible to this ratio of nutrients with the understanding that fluctuations of a few percent are normal.

The idea of practicality is definitely an issue with many people. When you are busy with work and everything else that crosses your mind throughout the day, you may not be as concerned with exact percentages and meal schedules. When you adhere to the schedule as strictly as mentioned above, you will get the best results. Begin with the nutritional requirements outlined in these chapters, and if you still have questions as to what is right for you, it is recommended you visit a nutritionist and seek professional advice.

Training: It's a Mental Thing

Focus on the journey, not the destination. Joy is found not in finishing an activity but in doing it.

— GREG ANDERSON

There are many different ways to exercise and train the body. Individual experts most likely have their own opinion and way of doing things they believe work best, but the truth is that there are a number of ways you can train your body to the get the most out of your workouts. What works well for one person might not be the best fit for the next. You may want to entertain several different strategies before you find one that is a comfortable fit for you. Depending on how active your everyday lifestyle is and what your interests and goals may be, you need to choose a plan that is realistic. Building a workout and nutrition plan that is balanced with your family life, work schedule, and interests is a smart way to go. With a little bit of thought and preparation, you can develop a plan that works for you.

If you work a job such as construction, you probably will not have to keep a rigorous training schedule. You should train moderately and pay attention to your nutrition. If you work in a cubicle and sit behind a desk all day, you will probably need a more intense workout regimen. People who have physically demanding jobs tend to be in better shape than those who sits behind a desk all day answering phone calls. If you fall somewhere in between these two examples, you will want to choose your fitness plan carefully. There are plenty of resources available to help you select the plan that meets your specific needs.

A solid exercise plan should consist of stretching, mental preparation, resistance training, cardiovascular work, and proper nutrition. As with anything else in life, balance and preparation will be the keys to your fitness success. Without these, you will see poor results and will not be able to reach your desired goal. Many people have begun a fitness regimen without balancing their lifestyle, nutrition needs, and workouts accordingly, only to say that it doesn't work. Do not fall into this category and become one of those people who give up before doing it the right way. If something is not working to your satisfaction, you should evaluate and fix the problem.

Excuses Anyone?

When a resolute young fellow steps up to the great bully, the world, and takes him boldly by the beard, he is often surprised to find it comes off in his hand, and that it was only tied on to scare away the timid adventurers.

— RALPH WALDO EMERSON

In order to be successful in your training, you have to want it. Doing it because your wife or husband told you to will not be enough. You need to feel the excitement and put some heart in it. Anyone who is successful in life did not get that way by just dumb luck. Luck would make for a great story, but the truth is that successful people have a plan for completing whatever goal they want to achieve. Luck is usually coupled with some desire and preparation. Even if it is not evident to those who are watching, people who achieve greatness have some sort of a plan and want to be winners. They may not admit this to you, but somehow the law of attraction is working in their favor. They must have dreamed of the outcome at some point in their lives and then took the necessary actions to make it a reality.

Do not let excuses hold you back. Excuses are so transparent and easy to come up with that most people can recognize right away that you don't have the guts to follow through with what you say you will. So, how does that make you feel? Here are a couple of reasons why people make excuses:

- They lack the initiative to start something.
- They lack the willpower to follow their dreams.
- They assume things should be handed to them.
- They are worried about what others think.
- They are lazy.
- They don't wish to be successful.
- They don't believe in themselves.
- They are afraid of the unknown.

If any of the above traits are representative of your personality, you may be in trouble. However, if one or more of these traits resemble an obstacle you face, you have the power to take control and make a change. Be a leader and own your fears. Only when you admit what your problems are can you do anything to change them. In fact, all of the excuses you can think of can be traced back to one of two things: fear and laziness. Fear is at the root of all your failures and is a powerful obstacle that holds you back from your true desires. Laziness is when you lack the initiative to take action. This doesn't just apply to fitness, but also to your financial success and any other goal in life you would like to achieve. The good news is that the rules are the same for everyone. So, what does this mean for you?

Realizing you are not the only one who suffers from this crippling trait should give you a sense of comfort. Since you know you are not alone, it should be easier to face your fear and anxiety head-on. You may believe that your inner issues are personal only to yourself, but in truth the rest of the world can identify with how you are feeling. Humans share a lot of the same fears and uncertainties. Whether you do it by yourself or with a group of people, success is yours for the taking. You do not have to go alone at anything in this world if you do not want to. Phone a friend or a family member who is willing to listen and help. If none are available, look to join a support group in your area. When it comes to fitness, there are several organizations and resources that offer help and support. There is no reason to be afraid anymore. The sooner you get started, the better you will feel.

Now that this stuff is out of the way, it's time to get to the good part—the "putting-it-together" and "how-to" part. It is not always pleasant to call people out when they are making excuses, but it has to be done. You need to snap out of fantasyland and get with the program. Being in the real world with real solutions will get you the real results you are looking for.

Keep Your Goals in Front of You

The first thing you should do when you wake up in the morning is recite the list of goals you want to accomplish and come up with a plan of how you are going to do so. Even better, you should start preparing the night before for what you want to accomplish today. Keeping your goals in front of you is a great way to stay focused. It allows you to keep your head in the game while creating new opportunities for reaching your desired level of success. Setting goals helps you create a healthy boundary around what is really important in your life.

While your fitness and financial success are important, you should also have a list of other goals and priorities. Your family should always be a top priority, as should your career. In the end, accomplishing your goals is not going to be fulfilling unless you maintain some balance and healthy boundaries. Family and career are important but are no excuse to neglect yourself. Performing effectively is operating efficiently. Your priorities are yours to choose, but do be reasonable in your endeavors. Instead of watching television all night before you go to bed, take some time to plan out the next day. Figure out what your workday will be like and plan appropriately. For example, you can do the following:

- Pack the kids' lunches and make sure their books and clothes are ready for school.
- Have all of your food ready and packed for work and the gym.
- If you use supplements, have them all packed and ready.
- Have an idea of when you are going to work out and plan your meals accordingly.
- Make sure you pick out your clothes for work and gym the night before.
- With traffic and weather in mind, plan for getting the kids to school and yourself to work on time.
- Take into consideration your significant other's plans for tomorrow, such as showering, breakfast, laundry, etc. Be ready in the shortest time possible.
- Set the timer on your alarm clock and coffee machine.
- Make sure you know where your car keys are when you want to leave.
- Have a plan for tomorrow night's dinner in case you are running late when you get home.
- Take some time to reflect about what went well today and what you can do better tomorrow.

- Take five minutes to read something inspirational and keep your morale high.
- Go to bed early if possible so you are well rested in the morning.

These are just a few of the things you could spend time doing the night before, rather than trying to fit them in when you are in a hurry and are not sure what you need. Planning ahead is simple to do and will save you a lot of time and frustration.

Create Good Habits

Begin to develop good habits to replace your bad ones. Get into the routine of eating healthy and working out. Healthy nutrition combined with exercise will have a synergistic effect. This will help your body adjust to the new demands you are putting on it. If you can, try to create a daily routine that will help keep you on track. If not, practice proper nutrition and exercise whenever you can fit it in. If you work out late one night and early the next morning, you'll be much better off than if you miss a workout entirely. As far as your nutrition goes, don't skip meals and be sure to plan out when and what you are going to eat. It will help you save time and will ensure you have the energy your body needs for a workout. Remember, no excuses—only results. Your own health and wealth are at stake, and success will not come without a little bit of work on your part.

Besides planning ahead to maximize your potential, you need to keep a few other ideas in mind. Being "FitEnomic" means thinking and looking at things differently than you did before. When it comes to fitness, there are three main phases that you will continue to cycle through each day:

1. 1.Pre-workout: This is anything and everything you do before your workout. It includes your workload for the day, your nutrition, the amount of sleep you had the night before, and knowing which muscles you plan on working out.

2. 2.Training: This is your workout regimen and plan in action. It includes what you do to stretch your limits and improve your health and body. Don't walk into the gym and just pick out your exercises as you go. You need to be prepared and walk in with a plan for what you are going to be doing that day.

3. 3.Post-workout/recovery: This is anything and everything you do after your workout. It includes your stretching, nutrition, sleep, hygiene, and preparing for the next time you visit the gym.

These are not new ideas or concepts, but they show you how you need to think in terms of your health. Thinking like this will help you to focus on your goal and stay committed. Your path to financial success and wealth depends on it. Everything you do for your health will set you up to be a bigger earner and potential big shot. You will improve your relationships, your potential to lead, and the influence you have everywhere you go.

More Mental Prep

There are many ways to train your body and mind for better health and fitness. Different things work for different people. It is true that the basic principles don't change much, but styles and methods of training do change and continue to evolve. There are experts out there who will be quick to tell you that their way is the best and only way if you want to see real results. As long as you apply yourself and work to make a change, you will. It really can be that simple. All of the people who claim to have the best workouts most likely have made great improvements to their own and other people's bodies. But what works for one person may not be what is best for you. You need to pick a program that you are comfortable with, that is safe, and that does not make false promises. This book covers the basics and gives you insight into different ways of thinking about your health and fitness. Most good workout plans are built from the basics; therefore, you are on the right track.

There is no need to argue about who does a better job at working out. Just make sure you eat well and exercise, and you will see results. Be glad you have so many different options to choose from. This means that whenever you get bored with one program, you can switch and start another. This is called muscle confusion. The idea of muscle confusion is to switch things up on a regular basis to keep your body guessing and yielding results. Please make sure that when you begin a program, you see it through to the end, without changing the designers' rules. They have spent long hours creating something for your benefit. You should approach each new plan with an open mind and follow the directions as outlined. If you don't like the plan, do not do it. You can always go online and look for another one. The FitEnomics website is updated on a regular basis to supply you with the latest and most relevant information in fitness.

You have likely heard stories from people who set out to try a new fad nutrition plan with a specially designed workout. After a few short weeks with no results, they begin to cry and say that it doesn't work. But are they sure? There can be several reasons why they are not experiencing the results they had hoped for. They may lack discipline, they might have cheated on their nutrition, they might have skipped some workouts, or they might not have stuck with it for longer than three days. This happens much more often than you think. Please, save everyone the frustration and follow through with a program once you select one. In reality, fitness plans don't fail people—the people fail to execute the plan. Unless you are injured and cannot physically work out, there is no excuse good enough to justify being out of shape.

When you begin your new workout, you are going to be a little sore. Do not let this prevent you from continuing. You need to pick yourself up and move forward to make progress. Anytime you subject your body to a new kind of stress, you are going to experience some growing pains. It is more like a dull, sore feeling that disappears after a few days. The more your body gets used to it, the less you are going to notice your muscles feeling sore. If you have worked out or played sports before, you know the pain will not last long. The good news is that you are starting to improve and strengthen your body. You should be proud and congratulate yourself on a brighter and more lively future the moment you begin.

Map It Out

Since you are starting to train for your future as a successful, wealthy, and healthy individual, it would be a good idea to make a map of where you are going. This is good for three reasons:

1. It will help keep you focused on the goals of your training.
2. It will become concrete evidence of what works and doesn't work for you.
3. Should you ever fall off the horse, you will have the blueprint for resuming your successful path to health and wellness.

Writing down your results will give you a sense of accomplishment. You can use your past experiences to help you make more progress in the future. By writing things down, you are keeping a record of what does and doesn't work for you. Hiring a trainer in the beginning is a great way to learn and make sure you are doing everything correctly, but only you will know your body the best. Your knowledge of health and fitness will grow as fast as you can see results. This also allows you to be experienced enough to eventually create your own programs, rather than always looking to someone else for advice.

Being able to introduce variety is definitely important. However, this should not be implemented until you have a solid understanding of fitness and your body. If you start off with the training wheels provided in this book, you will begin to build a solid foundation for years to come.

Supplements

Many people choose to use supplements when they exercise and get in shape. Supplements are a multibillion-dollar industry and have come a long way since they were first introduced many years ago. Numerous athletes and fitness competitors have been advocates for supplementation. The bodybuilding and fitness industry is a huge showcase for what some of these supplements have done for people. When you are more physically active than the average person, you need to take in more calories and nutrients. Even when you are trying to lose weight, supplementation can offer huge benefits. It is amazing how the body changes and improves with proper nutrition. Supplements do help and can offer huge advantages but are not required for you to get into shape. If you do not feel comfortable taking them, don't.

There is some controversy as to how well certain supplements really work. The ads in magazines can go into great detail promising positive results. Some of the results may not be typical of what the average person can expect, but it is hard to tell. Supplementation is meant to accompany a fitness program. If you don't maximize your training and fitness program, you'll find that the supplements will not be as effective. You can't just take a pill and expect to lose weight and build muscle. It takes effort. Since most supplements are not regulated by the Food and Drug Administration, there is some concern over safety and purity. With a little bit of common sense and research, you should be able to make a good decision as to which supplements are right for you. Here is a list of some of the most common supplements on the market today:

- protein
- amino acids
- creatine
- beta-alanine
- waxy maize
- nitric oxide boosters
- meal replacement powders
- weight gainers
- testosterone boosters
- vitamins and minerals
- appetite suppressants
- caffeine
- energy drinks
- fat burners

Whatever you decide to use is up to you. This book does not include recommendations for any companies in particular, but several resources are available to help you choose what is right for you. You can visit www.fitenomics.com to learn more information on this topic.

Calorie Management

Many nutrition plans start with a recommended intake of about two thousand calories per day. There is a huge difference between the right and the wrong two thousand calories. The right calories will help you burn fat and develop lean muscle mass, while the wrong calories will cause you to gain fat. Stay away from the wrong calories as much as possible; this cannot be stressed enough. The road to your success depends on intelligent food choices. Remember, it does not have to taste bad to be healthy. If you are still concerned about taste, go out and pick up a healthy cookbook or take a class. You will not be disappointed. The healthy and tasty food options are plentiful.

There are a variety of nutritional programs available for you to choose from. Some are free, and some cost money. For beginners, simply add or deduct calories from your daily intake. The typical amount to add to or deduct from your daily allowance is in the ballpark of five hundred calories, but that number can be cut in half. The easiest way to keep track of your weight is to step on the scale. However, this is not the most accurate method. The best way to keep track of your weight gain or loss is to use a tool known as a caliper. Calipers measure the amount of body fat you are carrying around by pinching your skin in predetermined areas. This separates the fat from the muscle and gives you a more realistic reading. The waist, back of the arm, and thigh are a few of the locations used for measurement. This tool can be purchased at the store or online.

You are most likely accustomed to using scales that tell you how much you weigh. Scales are not as accurate as calipers, because they don't measure whether you are losing or gaining fat or muscle. There is also the potential for experiencing a certain type of emotional drain when you step on the scale. Your weight has the tendency to fluctuate up and down, depending on what you eat and drink and how much fluid is excreted from your body on a daily basis. If you become obsessed with weighing yourself every day, you run the risk of going crazy over the minor changes. In this case, the mirror is a better indicator of your progress. If you look and feel better but have gained two pounds since your weigh-in ten hours earlier, don't pay it any attention. This is counterintuitive to what most people want to do, but it's important to know, as the scale is not an accurate indicator of your progress. If you tend to obsess about how much you weigh, do not step onto the scale. If it does not bother you to see your weight fluctuate up and down, you can still use the scale. Just keep in mind that it is not as accurate as the caliper.

During this adjustment period, you are aiming to create a more productive and wealthier you. It is good to be somewhat scientific in your approach, but it is not worth making yourself sick over. How you look and how you feel are great indicators of your progress. For example, if you have an idea of your ideal weight but are three pounds short of your goal, don't worry about it. Worrying is only going to cause you stress and make your goal appear more difficult than it really is. Stay focused on your progress. You may hit a plateau at some point, and this is normal. Do not get discouraged. Stick with what you are doing, and you will keep improving. Sometimes it is better to just take a look in the mirror and ask yourself, "How do I feel?" If you have been working hard and have not been making any excuses, you are going to be pleased with what you see. Remember, getting in shape isn't just about weight; it's about attitude, as well.

When you exercise to get in shape and lose weight, you may find that weight loss is not the immediate result. Depending on your body type, you may be the kind of person who builds more muscle. This is good, because muscle burns fat and increases your metabolism. By increasing your lean muscle mass, you are increasing your body's potential to burn off and eliminate body fat and excess calories. When beginning a weight-loss program, you may actually gain a few pounds before you lose them. Do not become concerned about this. Everyone's body reacts differently to exercise. Rest assured that you are building new muscle that will help you maintain a new fit and toned physique. Any muscle you add will help to reinforce all of your valiant effort to stay in shape and be more productive. Ultimately, the goal is to build more lean muscle mass. The more lean muscle mass you have, the more efficient your body is at keeping off unwanted fat and extra weight.

The Training Split

When you are ready to organize your workouts, consider using a training plan that includes a split. This involves working different muscle groups on different days to prevent overtraining. You want to make sure you give your muscles enough time to recover from one workout to the next. If you break down your body too much and do not give yourself time to recover, you can cause yourself to get sick or injured and you can inhibit your results. Since you are serious about your wealth and prosperity, take the appropriate time to rest before your next workout. Over time you will build up your stamina and be able to work out more frequently and for longer periods of time.

Working out three days a week is a good place for beginners to start. For the average person, the workout should last for about forty minutes to an hour and be moderate in intensity. There are programs available that call for exercising three times a week for a period of about twenty minutes, but these programs should be very high intensity and are not for beginners. You can gauge your fitness level by considering the amount of endurance you start and end with. If you work out for two weeks and do not feel challenged, you can probably increase your intensity and/or the number of days you are training. You should always exercise caution when you are training so that you do not overdo anything to point of injury. A little bit of soreness and fatigue are normal and necessary for progress. If it hurts, then stop and do something else or do not do anything at all. Only you will know how far you can push yourself during each workout.

There are several ways you can organize your routines when creating a split. Here is a list of the different muscle groups you will want to split up and train on different days (though keep in mind that only the basics are discussed in this book):

- chest
- back
- legs
- shoulders
- biceps
- triceps
- abs and core work
- cardiovascular training

These are the most basic muscle groups people think of when they train. You can group muscles together and train them on the same day, or you can split the muscle groups into specific training days. Deciding which route to go will probably come down to how much time you have to spend in the gym exercising. You may be more comfortable working out at home, simply because it saves you time. However you start to train will be completely up to you.

Cardiovascular training should be included at least twice a week in the beginning, though for those who are very overweight and out of shape, cardio training is recommended three to five times per week at varying levels of intensity. Beginners need to start out slow and work their way up. This will help to prevent injury and becoming overwhelmed with an onslaught of too much new physical activity. You want build up some stamina and ease into your resistance training. Something as simple as walking around the block a few times will be good to start. Walking is an excellent form of cardiovascular activity. Your heart is at the center of your body and has a very important job. It is the pump that supplies you with the blood and oxygen to function and carry out any and all physical activity. You need to be especially certain you take good care of it.

Cardiovascular training is a great warm-up before lifting weights and any kind of intense physical training. You need to make sure that you stretch out well before any kind of physical activity. Though most experts will advise you to do your cardio work before resistance training, some suggest doing it after. There are several schools of thought as to which one is right. Just make sure you fit it in somewhere in your routine.

Timing and Rest Periods

To help vary the intensity of your workouts, you should time yourself between sets with a stopwatch. Doing so will keep your routine fresh and challenging. Anywhere from forty seconds to two minutes is an acceptable range to allow yourself to recover. You should change the length of your rest periods every few weeks or so. Timing is a key element in creating "muscle confusion." Muscle confusion is the idea of changing your workouts on a regular basis so your body does not get too used to a workout. The more used to something your body becomes, the less it has to work at completing the task. Your body is smart and will always adapt. If your body begins to work less, something needs to be done to increase the workload and encourage new results. This is precisely why some people hit a plateau in their training—they are in desperate need of a change in order to further their goals. The body needs to be rechallenged.

As you become more advanced in your training, you may want to change things more often. If you keep using the same rest period every time you work out, you end up cheating yourself. To keep your body responsive, you must switch it up a little.

Timing yourself is also a great way to prevent yourself from talking too much during your workout. The gym tends to be a social environment, especially when the same people are there working out all the time. Do not get too social and ruin your workout. You want to make sure you stay on pace and keep the intensity up. If you pay attention, you will begin to see people who come to the gym every day but whose bodies never really seem to change. These are probably the same people who spend way too much time socializing and complaining about how they wish they could get in better shape eating junk food. Just because you join a gym does not mean that you are going to get in shape. You still have to practice some common sense and work toward your goals. By now you should know that things don't just happen for no reason.

Below are some examples of split routines. Nothing is set in stone when it comes to designing a fitness program, but you do need to have a starting point. Working with someone who has some experience in training others is recommended. When you first join a gym, you may be offered several free training sessions. This would be a great time to ask questions. The examples below include exercises that utilize the equipment found in most major health clubs.

Split #1

This is a routine you can do three days per week. You will hit all of the major muscle groups and begin to develop your cardiovascular endurance. For example, your routine could be split up between Monday, Wednesday, and Friday. Remember to stretch and warm up before any physical activity. The muscle groups and cardio are split up among the three days.

1. The focus is on chest, shoulders, triceps, abs, and cardio. Do a warm-up set, followed by three additional sets of ten reps. Fifteen minutes of cardio work should be done before or after your workout. Beginners should do about three exercises per muscle group including a warm-up set.

2. The focus is on your legs and abs. Since your legs include the largest muscle group in your body, you will need most of your energy to train them well. A warm-up set followed by three additional sets of ten reps will be sufficient. You should aim for about four or five different exercises for legs.

3. The focus is on back, biceps, and abs. Begin with a warm-up set, followed by three additional sets of ten reps. Fifteen minutes of cardio work should be done before or after your workout.

Monday	Wednesday	Friday
Chest, Shoulders, Triceps, Abs, and Cardio	Legs and abs	Back, Biceps, and Abs
Dumbbell Bench Press: 3 sets x 10 reps	Squat Machine: 3 sets x 10 reps	Seated Cable Rows: 3 sets x 10 reps
Triceps Cable Push-Downs: 3 sets x 10 reps	Lying Leg Curls: 3 sets x 10 reps	Weight-Assisted Pull-ups: 3 sets x 10 reps
Dumbbell Shoulder Press: 3 sets x 10 reps	Seated Leg Extensions: 3 sets x 10 reps	Alternating Seated Bicep Curls: 3 sets x 10 reps
Machine Ab Crunches: 3 sets x 25 reps	Hanging Leg Raises: 3 sets x 25 reps	Alternating Ab Crunches (side to side): 3 sets x 10 reps

Split #2

Before any kind of physical activity, you need to make sure you stretch and warm the muscles up properly. All workouts should include a fifteen minute cardio session before or after your resistance training. The three exercise routines are:

1. The focus is on chest and back. Begin with a warm-up set, followed by three additional sets of ten reps.
2. The focus is on arms and abs. Begin with a warm-up set, followed by three additional sets of ten reps.
3. The focus is on legs and shoulders. Begin with a warm-up set, followed by three additional sets of ten reps.

Tuesday	Thursday	Saturday
Chest and Back	Arms and Abs	Legs and Shoulders
Bench Press: 3 sets x 10 reps	Biceps Curls with Straight Bar: 3 sets x10 reps	Seated Leg Press: 3 sets x 10 reps
Seated Machine Rows: 3 sets x 10 reps	Triceps Push-Downs: 3 sets x10 reps	Squats: 3 sets x 10 reps
Incline Bench Press: 3 sets x 10 reps	Alternating Biceps Curls: 3 sets x10 reps	Leg Extensions: 3 sets x 10 reps
Lat Pull-Downs: 3 sets x 10 reps	Seated Dips: 3 sets x10 reps	Lying Leg Curls: 3 sets x 10 reps
Dumbbell Fly: 3 sets x 10 reps	Reverse Curls with Cambered Bar: 3 sets x10 reps	Seated Shoulder Press: 3 sets x 10 reps
One-Arm Dumbbell Rows: 3 sets x 10 reps	Lying Triceps Extensions: 3 sets x 10 reps	Dumbbell Lateral Raises: 3 sets x 10 reps

Split #3

Before any kind of physical activity, you need to make sure you stretch and warm the muscles up properly. This routine focuses a little more on stability and toning the muscles. The three exercise routines are:

1. The focus is on back, biceps, abs, and cardio. Begin with a warm-up, set followed by three additional sets of ten reps. Fifteen minutes of cardio work should be done before or after your workout.

2. The focus is on legs, abs, and cardio. Begin with a warm-up set, followed by three additional sets of ten reps. Fifteen minutes of cardio work should be done before or after your workout.

3. The focus is on chest, triceps, shoulders, and cardio. Begin with a warm-up set, followed by three additional sets of ten reps. Fifteen minutes of cardio work should be done before or after your workout.

Monday	Wednesday	Friday
Back, Biceps, Abs, and Cardio	Legs, Abs, and Cardio	Chest, Triceps, Shoulders, and Cardio
Lat Pull-Downs: 3 sets x10 reps	Seated Leg Press: 3 sets x 10 reps	Dumbbell Flat Bench Press: 3 sets x 10 reps
Seated Cable Rows: 3 sets x 10 reps	Walking Lunges: 3 sets x 10 reps	Seated Fly Machine: 3 sets x 10 reps
Standing Dumbbell Curls: 3 sets x 10 reps	Lying Leg Curls: 3 sets x 10 reps	Cable Push-Downs with V Grip: 3 sets x 10 reps
Seated Preacher Curls with Cambered Bar: 3 sets x 10 reps	Leg Kick-Backs: 3 Sets x 10 reps (each side)	Triceps Kick-Backs: 3 sets x 10 reps (each side)

Monday	Wednesday	Friday
Stability Ball Sit-Ups: 3 sets x 25 reps	Hanging Leg Raises: 3 sets x 10 reps	Stability Ball Shoulder Press with Dumbbells: 3 sets x 10 reps
Elliptical Machine: 15 minutes	Exercise Bike: 15 minutes	Walking on the Treadmill: 15 minutes (at 5% incline)

*Note: It is important that you keep track of your progress and write down what you do during your workouts. It is recommended that you keep a notebook with all of your progress cataloged in order according to date and include the time, exercises performed, sets, reps, and any increases or decreases in productivity. At the end of this chapter, you will find a chart that you use to help you keep track of your progress. Visit www.fitenomics.com for more information on this topic.

Stretching

Stretching is very important. It helps to warm the body up and prevent injury from strenuous activity. It also helps to cool the body down after a tough workout. If you do not properly warm up and stretch before exercising, you run the risk of hurting yourself and delaying your results. In order for you to reach your goals as quickly as possible, many things have to happen. Stretching is one of the very important pieces of the puzzle you do not want to skip or leave out. Some even believe that stretching can help to define and separate the muscle groups in the body, making them more noticeable in your physique. The bottom line is that stretching is extremely important and should not be left out during any fitness program.

Recovery

After being hard on your body, you need to take proper measures to replenish and revive yourself, and this is where eating right comes in. From the moment you finish working out, your body is starving for nutrients, even if you are trying to lose weight. Nutrient timing is critical to your success in health and fitness.

Before and after you work out are the two most important times you need to eat the right calories. Your meal before you work out should be high in protein and carbs. This is to help fuel your workout and ensure you will have the required energy to get the job done right. After your workout, you will also want to stick with the high-protein and high-carb plan. Exactly how much you need will vary according to your body type and what your goals are. This may be a good time to experiment with a pre-or post-workout supplement. If you are confident in your understanding of nutrition, you will be able to piece together the appropriate balance of nutrients to fuel your body. A general rule of thumb when you are trying to build lean-mass is to take in about one third more carbs than protein in a post-workout shake. Otherwise, you can visit your local health food store and ask someone who is knowledgeable in nutrition to help you pick out what is right for you.

If you decide you want to use supplements, you can try one of the many available. It is probably best to experiment with different kinds until you find one that you like. The more natural and organic the product, the better. Some supplements are going to have artificial sweeteners in them, so you will have to look around for a product that is made without them. This may be one of the cases where artificial ingredients are hard to avoid. Fortunately, more natural low-calorie sweeteners are becoming popular and are making their way into the products.

Something to keep in mind with nutrient timing is nutrient balancing. It can be easy to have a one-track mind when it comes to nutrition. The idea of nutrient balancing is covered in the nutrition section, but it is important enough to mention here as well. With all of the fad diets on the market, the idea of balancing your nutrients can get lost in all of the excitement. Some of these plans will involve a high-protein, high-fat, and low-carb diet. They may or may not stress the very important need for vegetables and greens. Although these diets may offer some results, they are not meant to be a blueprint for how to eat healthy.

What you need to eat before and after a workout differs from what you should be eating the rest of the day. The high-protein, high-carb meal would not be appropriate before bedtime, and the high- protein, high-fat, low-carb meal would not be appropriate before a workout. Introducing a large amount of greens into your diet is very important, as well. The vegetables and greens are meant to help balance the body's pH levels. When people try fad diets or bodybuilders cut weight for a contest, they have the tendency to push their bodies into a more acidic state, which can result in heartburn or indigestion. Most people would reach for an antacid at this point, hoping for some sort of relief. Instead of relying on a pill or medication to correct the problem, eating a balanced diet with lots of greens and vegetables can help to eliminate many of these issues. Drinking spring or mineral water with a high pH level is also very beneficial.

Sleep

Sleep is very important to the human body. It is recommended that you get about eight hours of sleep per night. It is probably rare for many people to get the full eight hours. The norm seems to be more around five to six hours per night. Either way, do the best that you can. The more you can get, the better off you are going to be and feel.

Sleep is also recognized to be a great immune booster and is the preserver of your youth and vitality. Have you ever seen someone who has been up all night without sleep? Sure you have, and the look on that person's face says it all. That same person will look much better after getting a good night's sleep. Think about how good you look and feel after a long, uninterrupted session of rest and recovery. There are not too many things that can beat it. When the body is sick and worn down, the doctor always recommends bed rest. Combine that with some solid nutrition, and you will be on top of your game.

Alternatives to Weight Lifting

If you would rather not lift weights, there are many other ways for you to still enjoy a good workout. Playing sports, doing yoga or Pilates, and dancing are a few examples. And playing with the kids, walking the dog, and cutting the grass are some simple ways to incorporate exercise into your day. For beginners who are very out of shape, the whole idea is to get them moving again and enduring some sort of physical activity. If two-thirds of the population are considered to be obese, there must be a large number of people who could use and benefit from some exercise. Sitting on the couch, watching television, and drinking beer will not help anyone get ahead in life. Actions must be taken.

Doing something as simple as parking in the back of the parking lot and walking up to the store will give you a few extra minutes of exercise. Taking the stairs in the apartment building or office will also help you to burn extra calories. Years ago, society did not have many of the luxuries it has today. There also were not as many obese people as there are today. Just because something is a luxury and makes life simpler does not mean it is a good excuse for being lazy.

Sports

Playing sports is a great way to get exercise and not even realize it. Participating in sports is a fun hobby that has a side effect of getting you into better shape. Running up and down the football field, basketball court, or soccer field is going to burn off a lot of calories and help tone your muscles. Factor in the desire you have to play well and win, and now you are pushing yourself even harder and burning off more calories.

Playing sports will also increase your endurance and energy levels. It would be very reasonable to say you will enjoy a more productive work day once you incorporate exercise into your routine. More productivity equals more money in several cases. This is a win-win situation for your wealth and prosperity. You can exercise your competitive nature to be successful while you are building a better body for yourself. Participating in a sport is something you can enjoy that is also good for you. The positive benefits will most likely spill over into several areas of your life.

You may have doubts about your athletic ability and be concerned that you cannot play sports. Football, basketball, soccer, rugby, baseball, volleyball, tennis, and racquetball are all very physical sports. You still have options to choose from that will not require you to run all over the place.

Maybe you would be interested in something that involves a little less running but is challenging and engaging—something you can play at your own pace and grow to love. Have you ever considered golf?

Golf and Fitness

Golf is a sport that may help you leverage your fitness efforts from below grade to well above the standard. It is a sport that can be participated in by anyone who wants to play it. With some sports, age may be factor in determining whether someone is equipped to participate. With golf, you can play as a little kid or as an old man. Here are ten benefits to playing the sport of golf:

1. It is mentally challenging.
2. It is physically challenging.
3. It has no age restrictions.
4. It can be played year-round.
5. It is a great way to get in shape.
6. It is a great way to relieve stress.
7. It is great for hand-eye coordination.
8. It is a great way to network and meet people.
9. It is played all around the world.
10. It is fun.

Golf is gaining a lot of recognition. It does not matter what your background is or where your current athletic skill and ability may be. It is a sport in which you can develop yourself by playing and learning at the same time. It is never too late to pick up a set of clubs, take some lessons, and play a round of golf. You may be surprised by what the sport can do for you.

This could be the gateway to your physical fitness and financial prowess. When you have a goal in mind, you have a reason to improve yourself. The psychology of fitness is just as important as the training and nutrition. Being able to leverage your fitness efforts will give you a huge advantage over someone who is exercising just because the doctor said to. Golf does not appear to be a very physical sport, but many golfers are realizing the benefits of lifting weights, cardiovascular training, and solid nutrition. By participating in a sport like golf, you are creating an outlet for success and personal development.

Aside from helping you get into shape, golf is a great way to network and meet interesting people. Many highly paid professionals and business owners play the sport. It has been said that, "The real business deals are made on the golf course, not in the office." Maintaining a healthy lifestyle will help you improve many areas of your life, not just one. Golf can act as a bridge between your fitness and business dealings, thereby increasing your chances of achieving success. You never know when an opportunity will present itself and propel you to the next level.

Dancing

Have you ever watched *Dancing with the Stars* on television? If you have, then you must have noticed the great physical shape the dancers were in. Practicing the dance moves, which the participants spend many hours doing, is an excellent way to get in a workout. The contestants who appear on the show and compete definitely leave the show in better shape than they were in when they started. Clearly, dancing is a very physical and fun form of exercise. You get the added benefit of learning how to move and communicate with your body in a sexy yet sophisticated way. Just think of what a few good routines could do for your social life. Dancing will get you out of your head and into your body.

The continuous motions are an excellent way to expend calories and tone your muscles. Most dancers are very athletic and enjoy firm bodies. Another added benefit is the increase in flexibility. When you learn a dance, you are trying out new moves, steps, and stretches and you are pushing your body to new limits. Thanks to your desire to have fun, you will be teaching yourself new ways to gracefully slide across the dance floor; to top it off, you will look good doing it.

Visit a local dance club in your area on a Friday night. If you don't know where to go, just ask around or look it up online. You may be surprised to see how many clubs and restaurants hold dance parties. Learning to dance gives you the added benefits of exercise, the expansion of your social circle, and better mind and body coordination. The next time you head out for a night on the town, consider learning a few extra moves to show off for that special someone. Not only will you be able to impress others with how well you can move and dance, but you also will be in much better shape because of it!

Pilates and Yoga

Pilates and yoga are also great workouts that can strengthen your body. These two forms of exercise are different from each other, but both seem to attract people in search of a more elegant and grounded approach. They do not involve much weightlifting or cardio but they do promote core strength and agility. Developing better control over your mind and body will provide you with a stronger sense of serenity and awareness.

If you have not ever watched the movie *Pumping Iron*, you may want to sit down and watch it one evening. The movie opens with bodybuilders Arnold Schwarzenegger and Franco Columbo practicing ballet on a running board. At first the whole scene seems like a joke and leaves you to wonder a bit; then the reality of what they are doing hits you. In order for these guys to compete on stage, they have to go through a posing routine that demonstrates their muscularity. In order to be better showmen, the bodybuilders decide to add some elegance to their posing routines.

Blending fluid motions with a massive muscular physique makes for an impressive show. Just having big muscles and a chiseled body is not enough. Being able to show it off in an effective and graceful way is much more impressive. It adds a certain depth that an otherwise brute individual may lack. It takes a certain amount of time and talent to master a graceful posing routine. Developing a symmetry between muscular development, posing, and balance, all while keeping your composure, is an accomplishment. This demonstrates that fitness is the complete package, not just a single and unbalanced discipline.

Pilates and yoga offer you a way to balance out your body without having to lift and train like a bodybuilder. It would still be wise for you to lift some weights and practice resistance training. In fact, it is strongly recommended that you practice some form of resistance training. However, training for core strength and coordination is definitely a step in the right direction. Incorporating all different forms of exercise would be the smart way to ensure your optimal health and fitness.

Benefits of a Health Club

You may be wondering whether you should join a gym or health club. After all, couldn't you just exercise at home? The answer is yes—to both. Working out at home is good for the individual who is very short on time or lives far away from any kind of health club. Some people just don't want to join a gym and may be a little turned off by the shared equipment. Either way, the choice is up to you.

Gyms do offer several advantages. For example, the gym is a high-energy environment that is geared toward stress relief. Going to the gym allows you to take a break in your day and do something for you. Everything you need to lift weights and work out properly is going to be at the gym. Rather than spending a whole bunch of money on home equipment that may not be as good, you can borrow the gym's equipment. Most of the machines and weights in the gym are going to be durable and commercial grade. The fact that other people are around offers you many advantages, including:

- There is always someone to ask for advice.
- The professional training staff offers a certain level of safety and assurance.
- The energy you feel from other people working out is contagious.
- Someone is always available to offer assistance.
- It is a great way to network and meet new people with similar interests.
- You never know what you might learn.
- It gets you out of the office and allows for some personal time.

Your gym and health club experience will be what you make of it. If you are not a shy, introverted, and self-conscious person, you should strongly consider joining a gym near you. If being around and interacting with the public is not your thing, then just stay at home and work out.

Weekly Progress Report

Date/Time	Exercise	Sets	Reps	Progress	Notes

*Note: Use this chart to track your progress.

10

Supplements and Testosterone Boosters

Don't measure yourself by what you have accomplished, but by what you should have accomplished with your ability.

— ANONYMOUS

There is no doubt that supplements, when used properly, can be effective, but you do need to be careful and practice some common sense. Sometimes, this takes a bit of research. When it comes to over-the-counter growth hormones and testosterone boosters, you should be very cautious. There are some people who are looking to gain an edge and will do just about anything to get it. This may be against their better judgment, but perhaps they feel the reward will be greater than the consequence.

How effective can an over-the-counter supplement be? People pay big money for good results. It is no secret that beyond testimonials, the value of something is reflected in its cost. How much money you pay for something is an indicator of the amount of time and research the company put into developing its product. If you are looking for the real deal, meaning a product that produces results and has some clinical research behind it, you can expect to pay a higher mount. Products that do not cost as much are not necessarily bad products, but you need to question why they are cheaper. Is it because they are less potent, cheaply made, or knock-offs? Maybe the company got a good deal and decided to pass the savings on to you, the customer. The company could have purchased the product in bulk in hopes of reselling it for profit. There are several different supplement retailers that are in competition with each other and want to earn your business. Be informed, and do the research before you spend your hard-earned money.

Supplements are not regulated by the FDA. How can you tell if what the companies say about their products is really true? Is the product safe? Supplement companies have a lot of freedom to choose what they want to put in their products. It is not a highly regulated industry, but third-party companies are testing more and more of the supplements on the market. It is an advantage for companies to include in their advertising that their product has some kind of scientific research backing its results and has undergone a third-party test for purity. This practice is beginning to catch on. Some products will work well for one person and have no effect on another. Stick with the basics to ensure you are buying a stand-up product. Protein, amino acids, creatine, carbohydrate drinks, and caffeine are a few supplement staples you should be familiar with. Always research a new product and use discretion when making a selection. If you are still unsure of what to use for your body type, consult a professional for guidance.

Growth hormone (GH) will make your muscles bigger but also will make everything in your body bigger and can cause some serious health issues. When Barry Bonds began slugging all of those home runs, there were a few different signs that suggested he had some help. The most notable was the sudden increase in home runs he was hitting that year. Next was the increase in his hat size. Barry Bonds's head had grown larger because of the same growth hormone that was increasing his muscle mass and strength. Growth hormone is not just for muscles; it is for everything in the body. There is a reason that hormone levels taper off after an individual goes through puberty and becomes a mature adult. The people who do experience an overproduction of growth hormone suffer from a disease called gigantism. This is not normal, and the life expectancy of such people is believed to be shortened. If this is what it does to the outside of your body, think about what is going on in the inside. However, there has also been a lot of research done about the positive effects. Many people who use supplemental GH products in their more mature years report looking and feeling younger. Therefore, hormonal replacement therapy may be something for you to consider.

Supplements may or may not work for you; you really won't know until you spend your money and try them out. If you are a healthy individual and want to experiment with certain supplements, please use some common sense and seek the help of a professional. Your body is a priceless machine that is unlike any other in the whole world. What you do to yourself can have lasting side effects. Some may be positive, while others may be undesirable. Always try to think ahead about what is really important to you and what you want to get out of this life.

Here is a scary fact that you may not have known: every person has tumors and cancerous cells in his or her body. For most people, they remain dormant, which means they are inactive and not harmful. Sometimes, however, these cells can become active in the body. They may be triggered by something you introduce into your system and begin to do you harm. If you introduce a hormone into your body that is not supposed to be there, you may inadvertently be triggering these dangerous cells to become active. Suffering from a terminal disease is no way to celebrate a few pounds of fat loss and muscular gain. However, these foreign substances may have nothing to do with a person becoming ill. The best advice is to use a reputable product from a reputable company. If you do not know where the product is coming from and who it is made by, you may want to look for something better known.

When you get down to it, you can argue that anything you put into your body is anabolic or catabolic, which means it has an effect on your body's muscle mass. Food is no exception, but at least it is the normal and natural approach. You may not get the development as fast as you want, but you will get results if you do it right. If your gains are based upon the introduction of a hormone booster, what do you think will happen when you stop taking it? Some people will keep what they gained, while others will lose it. It all depends on how your body responds. The only way to find out is to do it and see what happens. The more natural the path that you take to achieve the results you want, the more you are going to keep what you have worked for. When you are working out hard, however, supplementing with over-the-counter products is acceptable and quite common.

If you take a supplement and see results, you are going to be pleased. You may feel stronger and more motivated and be inspired to continue doing what you have started. Finding something that works well will definitely provide a big boost to your confidence. Beware of becoming a little too reliant on supplements, as you may forget that the key to lean muscle growth is the food you put into your body. You should not rely on supplements alone. Your body needs healthy food and calories to grow and repair itself.

Individuals who use hormones and chemicals can actually set themselves up to become somewhat dependent on the supplement or substance they are taking. Although this starts out to be only psychological, it can very well turn into a physical dependency. Talk to someone who has taken steroids or growth hormone before; he or she can tell you firsthand the psychological and physiological effects these substances can have. This can be extremely dangerous, not to mention very costly to your health.

The professionals who take the real stuff tend to do it with more caution and guidance. If you decide to take a cycle, it would be in your best interest to go to a doctor who could do some blood work. This way, you will able to see what is going on with your body and where you might be lacking or doing too much. Then you could order (from a doctor) what you would need to restore your levels to their normal range. This will help put your body into a prime anabolic state. It may take a little while for the effects to become obvious, but you will soon start to see and feel results. This is where the idea of cycling comes into play. Your body can only take so much, and since you are manipulating your hormone levels, you need to be very careful. Professionals take years—not just a couple of months—to develop themselves. (*Note: this book is in no way, shape, or form promoting the use of illegal substances.)

There is such a thing as hormone-replacement therapy. This usually involves more mature people who have visited a doctor and want to look younger, feel younger, increase their libido, and increase their strength and stamina. Again, this requires the help of an educated professional and will cost some money. Be very wary of the over-the-counter quick fix.

Besides taking hormone boosters, you can also take hormone blockers, such as an estrogen blocker. This will help to increase your body's natural levels of testosterone. It will also give your skin that tight and dried-out look that many bodybuilders like to have for a competition. Even in this case, you are messing with something that may have an unwanted side effect. Taking this blocker can also cause your joints to become stiff and dry. Cycling would still be required for this type of herbal supplement. There are supplements you can buy over the counter that may be beneficial. Many of them are going to be a form of an herbal supplement. Statistically, somewhere around 50 percent of all drugs are manufactured from a type of plant. Chinese herbs and holistic medicines have been proven to be of much benefit to many people. When it comes to your body and your health, be sure to seek professional advice.

There have been reports that steroids and prohormones can mess with people's sex drive and state of mind in general. As far as the attitude thing is concerned, if you are a jerk now, you will probably be a bigger jerk on the juice. It is what it is. How it may affect your sex drive is a different story. Some people may find that their sex drive decreases, leaving them unable to perform as usual. Others may experience an increased desire to ravish their loved one or anyone else they can get their hands on. You will not know how it is going to affect you until you try it—if that is a risk you are willing to take.

Anabolic steroids are illegal. If you get caught using or trafficking anabolic steroids, you can get in trouble with the law. They are categorized as a schedule III substance, which puts them in the same class as amphetamines, methamphetamines, opium, and morphine. Possession of any schedule III substance is punishable by law and can include a fine and/or prison sentence.

If you search the Internet, you will find several cases in which professional athletes have been stripped of their medals, trophies, and standings in the record books because of their use of anabolic steroids. People believe that using performance-enhancing substances is cheating. No one knows how long for sure, but the use of steroids and growth hormones has been going on for quite some time. There is a slim chance that everyone who has been using these substances will be caught or accused. Regardless of whether you use them or not, you still have to put in the hard work for the reward to be worth it. Food, training, timing, sleep, preparation, and willpower are all required in order for steroids to be beneficial. If you do not do things properly, you will end up wasting a lot of money and jeopardizing your health. Athletic-performance-enhancing hormones are not the magic pill, but when used correctly, they do have some benefits. The medical community uses steroids to treat sickness and disease every day. These drugs are considered to be legal. Prescriptions are written on a regular basis with much less ethical concern surrounding their effects on patients and their illnesses. Why is that? There is definitely a cloud of contradiction surrounding the use of steroids. In one situation, it is acceptable to use them, and in another, it is considered illegal and unethical. You will have to wait and see what the future holds.

Whatever you can achieve naturally will end up sticking with you much longer than what you do using a drug or supplement. You will look and feel better and will not be potentially messing things up by creating an artificial imbalance in your body. When you are young, it is easy for you to think you are invincible and will not be affected by poor judgment and decisions. There is always the right and the wrong way to do things. Just remember that you are going to be an older, more mature individual for much longer than you were a young and immature one. What you believe you can hide now will be much more obvious in the years to come. For some, this happens much sooner than later.

Most people are going to do what they want to do, regardless of the consequences; this is not a secret. You know your own desires and ambitions best. Just keep in mind that the actions you take now may not have an immediate effect, but they will have an effect. You may have to wait longer than you thought for the result to be obvious. Fitness is not something you can purchase off of the shelf. It is a collection of ideas, thoughts, and actions that are implemented over a period of time. Do not sell yourself short of reaching the goal line.

Become Familiar with Your Body

No matter what you do in life, there may be a moment when something happens and you need to respond right then and there. There will be no preparation, no warning, and no time to supplement or juice up; you will just have to physically respond. If you believe you need to take something to make you bigger, stronger, and faster, to give you more energy, or to motivate you to act, how will your body respond without anything? In other words, supplementing can be a good thing to do with many benefits, but you should want to understand how your body will respond in a stressful situation without anything to help pump you up. Your true energy and drive should come from a place inside you and not be dependent on an outside source. The essence of energy is tangible, but the results can be proven in real life.

Whether you are involved in an emergency situation or you are about to begin a monster workout, you need to be prepared. Firemen never know when a building is going to catch on fire, police never know when a criminal is going to use deadly force, the military doesn't know when and where the enemy will attack, and you never know if you are going to encounter a personal emergency yourself. That is why fitness is a lifestyle and not just something you do in your spare time or purchase off the Internet. You are preparing to be the best when the best is asked of you or needed from you. As you should know, being the best you can be all the time brings many rewards. GH, test boosters, steroids, and even caffeine are helpful while you are taking them because they create an enhanced response from your body. When you are not taking them, it is a different story.

When people discontinue their use of enhancing products, they may feel sluggish, not as strong, and even depressed. This is the body working to recover from the imbalance that was created during the use of these products. The hormone and chemical levels in the body need to balance themselves out back to normal. If you do not believe this to be true, just ask a doctor. Better yet, ask someone who has used a few cycles of steroids or prohormones. People who use steroids and prohormones need to go through what is called PCT, which stands for post cycle therapy. This is the process of aiding the body in getting its hormone levels back to normal and warding off any long-term side effects. People who use these products are creating artificially high levels of hormones in their bodies, which can permanently inhibit their bodies from producing their own. This creates a situation in which they will have to be dependent on the juice or a hormone not created in their own bodies. This negative side effect can last a lifetime, be very expensive, and cause many more problems in the future. It is probably a scary and stressful situation to experience firsthand.

Many people who do use these types of products are prone to building some level of addiction. They may not become addicted, but the possibility is much greater than if they were not taking anything to begin with. Protein and amino acids are much safer to supplement with. These are the basic building blocks that the body uses to build and repair itself. Creatine and caffeine are two other supplements that have become a staple in growth, recovery, and performance. Even caffeine can be addictive. You hear people say all the time, "I cannot start my day until I have my morning cup of coffee." For some people, that morning cup turns into five cups. These people may even develop intense headaches when they do not get their caffeine fix from coffee or another source. Hopefully you understand what the point is here. There is something to be said for those who know where they stand without the help of an enhancement product. Do you know where do you stand? This is a great example of how psychology plays an important role in your health and fitness.

Selecting the Right Supplements

There is an obvious attitude in society today when it comes to fitness and supplementation. Some of this may stem from inexperience, while another source of the problem may be a lack of concern. If the attitude could be summed up into one sentence, it would read something like this: if it is not going to hurt me right now, then I will be fine. People have become overwhelmed by all of the claims to gains that the supplement industry makes about its products. With the help of hypnotic vernacular and some fantastic marketing, gym enthusiasts are too eager to try something new without giving it any thought. Common sense needs to be practiced when it comes to supplementation.

There are a ton of companies out there that want you to buy their product. The supplement industry is a billion-dollar business. How many people do you know who make an educated decision about supplements and what they put in their body? Most likely, they base their decision on what brand seems to be popular and has the most name recognition. They probably experience an emotional high while fantasizing about their new body after seeing an amazing ad.

There are several companies that design and market a quality product that is safe and will help you produce results. There are also some companies that are just out to make a quick buck and don't care about your fitness success. Since the supplement industry is not regulated, it allows for a few fakers to enter the race. Figuring out what is best for you and your body type can be a complicated task, but do take the time to research and ask the appropriate questions. Supplements are a good thing and do help. It is always a good idea to ask your medical doctor for an opinion before you start a new training regimen. Keep in mind that not all doctors are going to know everything about fitness and nutrition. Bodybuilding, fat loss, and supplementation are an art form all their own. You may consider asking your fitness trainer, nutritionist, or chiropractor for an opinion instead. Fitness trainers, nutritionists, chiropractors, and herbalists are respected in their own right. There have been many novice athletes and bodybuilders who have spent years researching and experimenting to find the right path to perfect health and physical fitness. What works for one person may not work for another. Some trial and error is to be expected when determining what works best for you, but turning yourself into a lab rat is not recommended and can even be a bit dangerous. Quality is of the utmost importance when selecting the right product.

Keep in mind that all of this information is open to debate. The supplement industry would not have lasted as long as it has if it did not offer any advantages. The key to picking the right supplements is doing your research and exercising some common sense. Here is a list of questions you should ask your-self when making your decision as to which supplement regi-men is right for you:

1. Do I have any preexisting conditions that may compli-cate my health?
2. Have I checked with my health-care provider, fitness trainer, and nutritionist before starting a new fitness routine?
3. How long has the company in question been in business?
4. Does the company's ad include real scientific data to back up its claims?
5. Does the company use quality ingredients in its prod-uct line?
6. Have I taken the time to research the product online?
7. If reviews are available, have I taken the time to read them?
8. What is it exactly that I am trying to accomplish?
9. If I am considering taking more than one supplement, what will work well together?
10. Is there anything I should avoid taking with my supplements?
11. Will these supplements affect any of the medications I am taking?
12. Am I willing to try to stick with a supplement regimen for a prolonged period of time?
13. How much money am I willing to pay for my supplements?

If you feel you still have some unanswered questions, give the company a call and ask to speak to someone who knows about the products. Make sure you get someone who under-stands health and science and who is not just a salesperson. The company may have the best product around, but if you talk to someone who is not confident about the product, you will definitely be able to tell. If it is a good company, smart and educated people will be available to answer your questions. If not, then choose another company with better representation. For more information on supplementation and what may be right for you, visit www.fitenomics.com.

Targeting one goal at a time will help to keep things less confusing. For example, if you are trying to lose weight, focus on weight loss rather than muscle development. If you are looking for dense muscle mass, focus on building your body rather than trying to stay lean. If you are more of an experienced athlete, you can combine your goals; this is assuming you are more knowledgeable about how to execute your program properly. If you are a beginner, in time you will understand how your body responds and can then take on more of a challenge. Training and supplementation are skills best developed cautiously. They are not something you want to risk doing wrong. Please make sure to consult an expert if you have any further questions.

11 Alternative Therapy

The art of healing comes from nature, not the physician. Therefore the physician must start from nature, with an open mind.

— PHILIPUS AUREOLUS
PARACELSUS

Society has become very impatient. People believe there can be a quick fix for everything and they do not have to wait for it. Whether the media or clever marketing is to blame for creating the "now" monster, things have changed, and there is definitely a strong driving force behind getting and wanting things faster. For example, fast food allows you to eat a hot meal within minutes, accelerated school programs allow you to finish your education faster, and technology has forever decreased the amount of time it takes for information to be exchanged and traded. Of course, there are always exceptions to the rule. When it comes to fitness, the faster and quicker method is not always the best choice for getting the job done right. There may be ways to speed up your results, but be careful not to sacrifice healthy gains.

It is true that technology has increased the rate at which people can make improvements and changes in their lives. The information is easier to find, medical education has evolved, producing more highly skilled and trained professionals than before, and the understanding of nutrition has developed in leaps and bounds. There are also a lot more options available today than there were in previous years. With an overload of information available at your fingertips, it can be hard to determine what is useful and what is garbage.

Have you ever read or heard the words "perception is reality"? Most likely you have. If you do not remember, keep reading and it should start to sound familiar to you. This great concept has been followed by many people who wished to get ahead in life. They realized they had the power to avert negative outcomes with their own positive way of thinking and feeling. This doesn't just apply to your own health, but also to any and every other thing you want to do with your life.

The Power of Thought

Instead of waiting for something to go wrong with your health and fitness, make sure you take care of yourself. Do not take for granted all of the things you can do without issues or concerns regarding your health. Walking without help, eating meals on your own, driving your own car, bathing yourself, and being of sound mind to make your own decisions are just a few examples. Everyday activities may sound simple, but without your health, they are quite difficult tasks. At some point, everyone will reach a stage in life where things are just more difficult than they once were. There is no reason to speed the process up and experience those days sooner than you have to. Everyone ages and gets older. It is up to you to take care of and harness your youth while you still can.

Stay mindful of your fitness and financial outlook in life. Keep your goals and motives in front of you and do not let them fall behind you. Even if you were dealt more of a difficult hand than someone else and you have an ailment you were told you have to live with, do not focus on it. Sure, it can be a bit of a challenge, but aim to make the best of it. The choice is yours—and only yours—to make. You have the power to prevent any negative thinking that could possibly hold you back from doing what you want to do. Nothing can make you feel bad unless you give it the permission to do so. As long as you say so, it cannot have an effect on you. You were created special, and you have the ability to free yourself from negative thinking. Even if a doctor has given you a poor prognosis, you do not have to accept the doctor's outlook about *your* future. Remember, don't believe anything too much. There is always an exception to the rule, and in this case, *you* can be the exception to the rule.

People who are diagnosed with disease do not have to give in to the fearful thinking that may be associated with their prognosis. There are true stories of people who were diagnosed with terminal illnesses, such as cancer, and completely beat the disease and healed themselves. People have made the decision to overcome the odds and live normal lives, no matter what. Doctors and scientists are not sure how it happened, but they are living proof. Others have been hurt in accidents and were told they would never walk again. They too beat the odds and are now able to walk. If you believe in something enough and set your mind to it, you can make the outcome you visualize your reality.

Be careful what thoughts you let sit and grow in your mind. Imagine that your mind is the most fertile farming ground in the universe. Each thought that you have is like a seed that is being planted for the future. Your mind does not know the difference between good or bad; it just makes sure that whatever you plant will have what it needs to grow. Based on this example, how important do you think your thoughts are? You need to be sure that you are only planting healthy and positive seeds and avoiding those things that are bad for you. If you plant something negative, it will show up and bring you grief. To avoid this, make sure your thoughts are positive and are focused on the good you want in your life.

Chiropractic Treatment

Chiropractic therapy offers an alternative to traditional medicine. There is definitely a time and a place for being treated by a medical doctor. You will need to do what is comfortable for you, but understand that you do have options. A chiropractor can offer you the possibility of receiving care without drugs and surgery.

Balance and homeostasis are the focal points of alternative medicine. Remember, everything in your body is based upon a pH balance. If something is out of line, you risk the possibility of suffering in some way, either physically, mentally, or socially. An adjustment will need to be made.

When you seek medical attention, your doctor will offer a diagnosis. You may be prescribed a medication, some pain pills, or nothing at all. You may be told that simply eating better and getting more sleep will be sufficient. But there may be a time when no matter what you do, the problem does not seem to get any better. You may become more worried and stressed out from dealing with all of the tests and uncertainty surrounding your ailment. So, what is an acceptable alternative?

Chiropractors are ready and willing to provide you with peace of mind and alternative therapy. In a professional and educated manner, they can offer you medical advice that can make a huge difference. Chiropractic therapy helps to relieve nerve disruption and recreate the free flow of energy you once enjoyed throughout your whole body. If you have a block somewhere or something is out of line, a chiropractor can restore your body to the original state it was in so that you can begin healing. The outcome is different for everyone. Some people become more relaxed, while others feel restored and have more energy.

Many sports professionals use chiropractors on a regular basis. You probably have a friend or neighbor who has had an experience with one. It is all right to be a little hesitant about getting adjusted. Fear of the unknown is what keeps many people from enjoying a much higher quality of life. Your health and happiness are worth the time it would take to research this type of therapy. If you have any questions or concerns about chiropractic therapy, you should visit with a professional. Do not, under any circumstances, let someone who is not licensed adjust your back. Although it appears to be an easy thing to do, it is not worth suffering an injury at the hands of someone who is not properly educated. Chiropractors have gone to school for several years and are licensed doctors in their profession. They take their work very seriously. Many times, they will work with your family doctor to make sure you are getting the best care possible.

Using the Sauna

The sauna is a great way to heal your body. Not everyone is comfortable sitting in a very warm room just to sweat, but doing so can be very good for you. Sweating serves a few different purposes for the body. It is the mechanism the body uses to cool itself down when it is too hot. It is also a way for the body to shed and release toxins. Showering after using the sauna is a good practice to get into. This helps to wash away whatever substances your body was trying to get rid of, rather than letting them be reabsorbed.

It is true that you lose other nutrients the body needs when you sweat; that is to be expected. To ensure that you are using the sauna safely and properly, you should check with a health-care professional to see if you have any restrictions. Next you should abide by all of the rules associated with sauna use. Practicing good personal hygiene is a must. Before you sit in the sauna for any amount of time, make sure that you are properly hydrated. You should drink copious amounts of water before and after using the sauna. Practicing proper nutrition is also a good idea if you are going to be an avid sauna user. You do not want to dehydrate yourself and become sick.

The sauna can be overused and abused if not properly monitored. Setting a time limit before you enter will help you avoid staying in for too long. If you need to walk out and take a break, do not hesitate to do so. The sauna is also used by people who are looking to lose weight. Wrestlers and martial arts practitioners are known for wearing sweat suits and sitting in the sauna. This helps them to cut weight before an athletic event weigh-in. The weight they lose is mostly water and will be gained back quickly. These athletes are usually supervised by a trainer and know what they are doing. Do not use the sauna as a quick-fix solution for losing weight. It is not healthy and strongly advised against. Please exercise caution if you decide to use the sauna. It can do you some good when used properly in small amounts of time.

Detoxification

There are many ways to detox your body. You can follow a special nutrition plan designed for cleaning out your body or you can purchase a detox supplement from your local health-food store. There is some speculation as to how effective detoxifying your body can be. Many people have experienced some positive results. Some of the benefits you may experience after a successful detox include:

- Weight loss
- Better digestion of food
- Higher energy levels
- More restful sleep
- Sense of well-being
- Improved attitude and outlook

Be sure to consult a health-care professional before performing a detox on your body. You want to make sure that you do not do anything that will conflict with any medications you may be taking. If you do have a clean bill of health, be sure to choose a reputable supplement or detox plan. Your local health-food store may be a good place to start. Hopefully, the person working behind the counter will be knowledgeable and can offer you some helpful advice. Otherwise, asking your doctor or chiropractor or using the Internet would be your best bet. Holistic medicine is another option you may want to consider. You should choose a reputable practitioner with a strong track record of helping and healing people.

12
Develop Your Mind Set

I think and think for months and years.
Ninety-nine times, the conclusion is false.
The hundredth time I am right.

— ALBERT EINSTEIN

This section of the book has been included to give you some additional motivation and inspiration. Similar to an affirmation, the ideas here are meant to be encouraging and keep you focused on the greater prize at hand. Fitness is only one component of your health and wealth, but it will be your vehicle for transforming into the person you wish to become. The next few pages can act as a catalyst to help push you over any sticking point you may encounter along the way. You are encouraged to come up with a few affirmations of your own.

Statistics will show that words are 7 percent of communication, while tone of voice and body language make up the other 93 percent. However, the words you use to communicate with yourself hold a little more weight than 7 percent. Words do influence and hold tremendous value when accompanied by feelings and leveraged with a goal in mind. From the moment the thought is first conceived and before it can even be put into words, it is automatically linked to emotions and intelligence. This influence helps construct and formulate an idea to be communicated. You must communicate the idea with yourself before you can share it with anyone else.

Your line of thinking, whether positive or negative, will project a certain energy to the idea before it can be implemented and carried out. With that said, use this section to practice communicating with yourself in a positive way. Thoughts become things, and when you focus in the right way, you give yourself the power to accomplish anything you wish. You must understand this principle in order to be successful and have a winning attitude. Your positive or negative thoughts are like a special code for your mind that generates the results you will experience in your life. Make sure you are programming the right code and staying on a path of growth and fulfillment. The information here should be used as a guide to further develop your own goals and motivations so that they can take root.

HEART

Heart is a force that drives, inspires, motivates, captivates, heals, and loves. To many it is felt, to some it has to be seen, and to all it is recognized. It is a guide for those who are looking for more than what they are currently receiving or delivering. It is not just about one but about many who are alive and want to feel more. It goes with you wherever you go and is always an available resource to call upon. Stretch your potential, play for keeps, and create memories that make life worth living. What you create now has the potential to affect many who follow in your footsteps.

Your attitude is everything. Live your truth. You are telling the world how you live, play, and love and how you look at any situation you encounter. When a situation gets tough and things are not the way you would like them to be, the amount of heart you carry with you will be evident. You are either going to be the kind of person who will quit or you are going to embrace your inner strength and believe you will become whoever or whatever you need to be in order to be successful and live a happy life.

PLAY

It is possible to always feel youthful. Remember, age is a mind-set. How you view yourself in this world says a lot about your self-worth and how others will view you. Confident people have a way about them that is contagious and coveted by others. Their presence is reassuring and inspiring. Add a touch of class and a hint of charm, and you will have a recipe for boosting anyone's self image.

Life is about learning and becoming. You should not be a static being who just sits still and waits for things to happen.

Your goal should be to do, rather than to react. Just as you have your good days, you also will have some bad days. You need to have the bad in order to recognize the good. Each morning when you wake up, you can decide which way to take your life. Every decision you make today will shape your tomorrow. Choose wisely.

POWER

Becoming the master of yourself and your abilities is an outstanding feat to accomplish. Consistently working to improve your mind and body can bring you a level of happiness that will last a lifetime. Harness your energy, increase your potential, and set your sights on what you want to achieve. As long as you employ your own personal power, you stand to be an unstoppable force.

It has been said time and time again that anything is possible if you put your mind to it. You become what you think about. The only way you can do something is if you give yourself the permission to do it. You need to trust yourself and not look to someone else every time you have a problem to solve. What is right for one person may not be what is right for you. Free yourself from the grasps of others and learn to rely on your own intuition. It was given to you for a reason.

STRENGTH

You possess power within in you. As an individual you are strong, but when you are part of a team, you are stronger. There are strength in numbers and anything is possible. The greatest achievements did not result from a single person doing a job, but from several people working toward the same common purpose. Whether you and your team are in the spotlight or not visible at all, you are building a bond that can carry and unite you.

FOCUS

When you make up your mind to do something right, there is not much that can stand in your way. You will be able to block out any negative influence and tune into your dreams and desires. To be focused is to firmly embrace the idea of success. There is no other way. You are entirely tuned in to your goal and will bring your belief and creation to life. Others will take notice of this positive trait you possess and be drawn to you.

FATE

You may not understand why things happen the way they do. You may even feel like you are going in reverse and not making any progress. Stay strong and continue on your path to personal development. You are growing as an individual and will experience what you must to surpass your current state of being. Act as if your goal has already come to pass, and it will be purposefully attracted to you.

REACH

When you first step out of bed in the morning, know that the day ahead of you is yours to conquer and make your own.

Successful people got where they are by making the decision to rise above the rest and reaching out to further their talents, dreams, and desires. Most people would call these talents gifts, but the truth is that they came from hard work and practice. Achieving goals requires a tremendous amount of effort. Those who understand this know they have a certain amount of time to get things done and do not waste the opportunity. They tell themselves they can do it, they give themselves the permission, and they don't allow anything to stand in their way. Be honest with yourself about what you really want and commit yourself to doing whatever it takes.

LIVE

You know that feeling when you are on to something
　　great,
Whether awake or dreaming, you are sealing your fate.
You may look over your shoulder but focus ahead,
Listen to your desires and you will be led.
Don't live in the past, the present is here,
Being present in the moment is nothing to fear.
You will guide, not judge; don't cry, just love
Thoughts that were cloudy before will now become
　　clear.
It is up to you, it always has been,
For now and forever, there is no end.

LOVE

To many it's more, to some it's less—
Like a leap of faith, just hold your breath.

To know is to be seen, to be seen is to be heard,
Others around you will listen to the power of this
     word.
So deeply it is felt that open wounds it will cure,
It washes away all madness, it's essence is so pure.
Think of a beautiful nature scene,
Undisturbed and untouched, like the ones in your
     dreams.
So perfect, so clear, whether far or near,
It seems so close, it is always right here.
It cannot be captured but is held loose and free,
No strings of attachment, but it binds you happily.
It brought you here in the beginning and will be there
     in the end,
It is always around you it comes from within.

LAUGH

What is that sound you can hear from afar,
It can show up in an instant wherever you are.
Whether here right now or later on maybe then,
When it comes it's contagious and you'll do it again.
It picks you up when you are down and it will help
     you outlast,
All that was wrong is now right whenever you laugh.

Although this book may be over, do not think of this as
an ending. Use the information here as inspiration for you to
change and take your life in a new direction. You may already
be living a good life. Why not live a great life? Many people
who are on top of their game can credit a mentor or coach to
help keep them in line and on track. This is your opportunity

to find that inspiration and play the game that much better. Be inspired, live life to the fullest, and expect only great things to come from this point on. God bless!

You can learn more at <u>http://www.fitenomics.com</u>.

References

Brand-Miller, Jennie, Joanna McMillan-Price, Katherine Steinbeck, and Ian Caterson. 2009. "Dietary Glycemic Index: Health Implications." *Journal of the American College of Nutrition* 28:446S–449S.

Gleeson, M., and D. C. Nieman. 2004. "Exercise, Nutrition, and Immune Function." *International Journal of Nutrition and Exercise Metabolism* 22:115–125.

Kanter, M. 1994. "Free Radicals, Exercise, and Antioxidant Supplementation." *International Journal of Sports Nutrition* 4:205.

Lemon, P. W. 1998. "Effects of Exercise on Dietary Protein Requirements." *International Journal of Sport Nutrition* 8:426–447.

Marieb, Elaine Nicpon, and Katja Hoehn. 2012. *Human Anatomy and Physiology*. Ninth edition. San Francisco: Benjamin Cummings.

Robbins, Anthony. 1987. *Unlimited Power*. New York: A Fawcett Columbine Book / Ballantine Books.

Schwarzenegger, Arnold. 1993. *The Education of a Bodybuilder*. New York: A Fireside Book / Simon & Schuster.

Society of Actuaries. 2011. "New Society of Actuaries Study Estimates $300 Billion Economic Cost Due to Overweight and Obesity." Press release.

Tipton, K. D., and R. R. Wolfe. 2001. "Exercise, Protein Metabolism, and Muscle Growth."

International Journal of Sport Nutrition and Exercise Metabolism 11:109–132.

Tsintzas, K., and C. Williams. 1998. "Human Muscle Glycogen Metabolism During Exercise:

Effect of Carbohydrate Supplementation." *Sports Medicine* 25:7–23.

United Nations Development Programme. "The Millennium Development Goals." http://www.undp.org/content/undp/en/home/mdgoverview.html. Accessed on July 20, 2012.

United States Department of Agriculture. "Food Groups Overview." http://www.choosemyplate.gov/food-groups. Accessed on July 20, 2012.

Zawadzki, K.M., B. B. Yaspelkis, and J. L. Ivy. 1992. "Carbohydrate-Protein Complex Increases the Rate of Muscle Glycogen Storage after Exercise." *Journal of Applied Physiology* 72:1854–1859.

———. 2000. "Beyond the Zone: Protein Needs of Active Individuals." *Journal of the American College Nutrition* 19:513S–521S.

About the Author

Ryan Weber works full-time as a fire fighter/paramedic and has been a certified fitness trainer. He is also a nationally qualified fitness competitor in the National Physique Committee (NPC) and competes in the men's physique division. His passion for fitness and helping others offers an outside-of-the-box approach to living and maintaining one's well-being. Having been raised in a health-conscious family with a medical background, he demonstrates with purpose that healthy living is essential for a life of happiness and prosperity.